Yoga Wheel

Selina Reichert

YOGA
WHEEL

**102 Poses to Improve
Strength, Balance,
and Flexibility**

Meyer & Meyer Sport

British Library of Cataloguing in Publication Data
A catalogue record for this book is available from the British Library

Yoga Wheel
Maidenhead: Meyer & Meyer Sport (UK) Ltd., 2025
ISBN: 978-1-78255-274-1

© 2025 by Meyer & Meyer Sport (UK) Ltd.
Aachen, Auckland, Beirut, Cairo, Cape Town, Dubai, Hägendorf, Hong Kong, Indianapolis, Maidenhead, Manila, New Delhi, Singapore, Sydney, Tehran, Vienna

CREDITS
Cover and interior design: Anja Elsen
Layout: DiTech Publishing Services, www.ditechpubs.com
Cover photo, section photos, and chapter photos photographer:
Andrius Tekorius – Photographers in Fuerteventura & Lanzarote
Cover and interior photos: All rights remain with the publisher
Managing editor: Elizabeth Evans
Copy editor: Sarah Tomblin, www.sarahtomblinediting.com

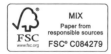 Member of the World Sport Publishers' Association (WSPA), www.w-s-p-a.org

Printed by Print Consult GmbH, Munich, Germany
Printed in Slovakia

MIX
Paper from responsible sources
FSC
www.fsc.org
FSC® C084279

ISBN: 978-1-78255-274-1
Email: info@m-m-sports.com
www.thesportspublisher.com

CONTENTS

PREFACE

Dear yoga friends!

It is with great pleasure that I share this book to take you on an inspiring journey with the Yoga Wheel. It is my heartfelt wish to meet each of you, whether beginner or advanced, regardless of age, at your individual level and lead you to new challenges for body, mind, and soul.

The easy-to-understand exercises in this book are suitable for beginners and advanced practitioners alike. Through regular practice and the conscious execution of the breath, these exercises offer a unique opportunity to challenge yourself on different levels. The aim is to develop a deeper awareness of the body and improve the ability to relax.

Similar to my yoga classes, this book takes you through the warm-up phase with the Sun Salutation to various poses with the wheel—from standing to floor exercises. Some exercises do not yet have an established name, so I have given them their own new names.

Take your time with the individual exercises and be patient with your body, the Yoga Wheel, and yourself because they need to get to know each other first. For further inspiration, I invite you to try one of my workshops or intensive courses. Content me through my website, and I can provide instruction in English: www.yogaandpoleartbyselina.com.

I wish you a wonderful time trying out and discovering. May this journey lead to more joy, serenity, and self-development.

Namaste,
Selina

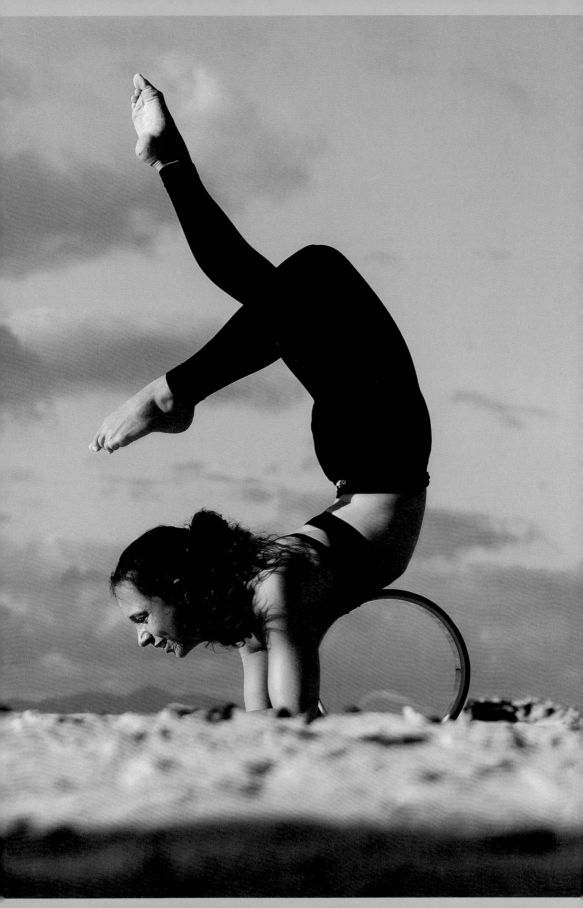

ACKNOWLEDGMENTS

This dedication is to my wonderful volunteer supporters who have accompanied me on every page of this book journey.

An especially heartfelt thank you goes to my best friend Janine from Frankfurt am Main, who generously agreed to take the beautiful photos of me for this book during our vacation in Greece.

Another sincere thank you goes to my uncle Klaus, an established author in Germany, who always gave me words of encouragement. His support has inspired me not to give up on my book idea and to believe that this work will eventually be published beyond the borders of Germany.

I would also like to take this opportunity to thank my mom, Lorena, who sadly passed away from cancer in 2023; she was a true sporting inspiration and role model. She supported me unconditionally in all my sporting goals, be it pole sports or yoga, and paved the way for my own sporting journey.

And last but not least, my thanks go to my valued course participants who welcome me every week with openness, curiosity, and motivation. Witnessing your successes is a precious moment of happiness that I would not want to miss. Your trust gives my journey as a trainer a deep meaning.

Thank you and Namaste.

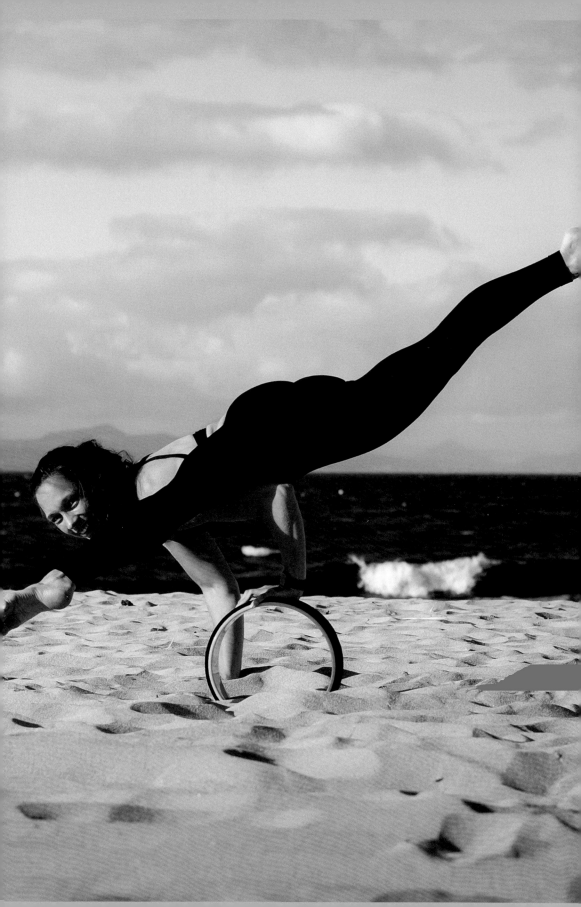

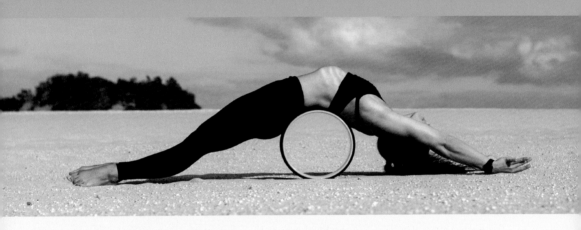

INTRODUCTION

THE YOGA WHEEL

The origins of the Yoga Wheel, also known as the Dharma Yoga Wheel, reach deep into the centuries-old history of yoga. This unique tool has its roots in the original intention to support yogis on their path to achieve advanced asanas and deepen their practice.

Visionary American yoga teacher and engineer Sri Dharma Mittra has combined this ancient practice with contemporary innovation to create the Yoga Wheel. With his years of experience in yoga and his deep understanding of engineering, he wanted to develop a tool that would support yogis at all levels of experience. The wheel was designed to promote flexibility, improve balance, and stretch the spine.

The idea was born out of a desire to help yogis in advanced asanas while making the practice more accessible to beginners. Dharma Mittra founded the company Dharma Yoga Wheel, which specializes in the production and distribution of these aids. Since its introduction, the Yoga Wheel has gained popularity worldwide and is now a commonly used tool in the yoga community.

Available in different materials and designs, from plastic to elegant wood, the diameter usually varies between 30 and 35 cm (12 and 14 in), with a width of around 12–15 cm (5–6 in). Many wheels are equipped with a soft, non-slip coating that ensures a secure grip during intensive exercises.

The variety of materials allows for different load capacities, often between 150 and 200 kg (330 and 440 lb), depending on the manufacturer's specifications. To vary the exercises, one or two yoga blocks can be used as an elevation aid or to fix the bike in place to make it easier to perform the exercises. The nature of the block, whether it is made of cork or hard foam, influences its load-bearing capacity.

Today, the Yoga Wheel and yoga block are easily available on the internet or from sports retailers. Their wide range of applications make them valued companions in yoga practice, and their use enriches the yoga journey with joy, ease, and perhaps also spirituality. Immerse yourself in the world of the Yoga Wheel, and find out how this simple but effective tool can enrich your yoga journey.

MORE ABOUT THE YOGA WHEEL AND ITS ADVANTAGES

The Yoga Wheel, a versatile aid, opens up a world of relief and challenge in your yoga practice, not only for beginners but also for advanced practitioners. For beginners, the wheel acts as a supportive tool that makes it easier to hold certain yoga positions for longer. An example of this is its use as an elevation in Warrior variations or to relieve pressure on the shoulders and back during Forward Bends.

For advanced practitioners, the Yoga Wheel makes it easier to hold balancing poses, gradually strengthening muscles and coordination through regular practice. The wheel also supports the stretching and elongation of the thigh muscles and hips. The right breathing technique can also open up and strengthen the chest, shoulder, and back muscles.

Tension and blockages in the back can be released during training with the Yoga Wheel, resulting in improved mobility and relaxation. Heart-opening poses in particular, such as Backbends and forearm balances, are encouraged by the Yoga Wheel and take on a new dimension.

The Yoga Wheel also serves as an effective strengthening device for the core. Numerous exercises for the back and abdominal muscles can be performed using this tool, resulting in holistic strengthening and improved posture. Immerse yourself in the world of the Yoga Wheel and discover how this simple but effective device can enrich your yoga practice.

HOW DO I COMBINE INDIVIDUAL EXERCISES?

To create a harmonious yoga flow with the Yoga Wheel, it is important to master the basic seated, standing, and lying poses as well as various stretching and strengthening exercises. Start your practice with gentle warm-up exercises to prepare the body. Structure the flow so that you gradually increase the intensity by moving from basic exercises to more advanced poses. However, only do this if you feel confident in the individual poses and can perform them cleanly.

Make sure that the transitions between the individual exercises are smooth and avoid abrupt changes. If you feel unsure in some asanas, use aids and continue to practice them as individual elements.

Coordinate the movements with your breathing to create a meditative atmosphere and support the flowing transitions. Conclude the flow with calming and relaxing exercises using the Yoga Wheel for support. After you have completed the flow, reflect and make a note of which asanas worked well and which you would like to work on, and perhaps even create your next flow. The key lies in the intuitive design, which is based on the individual needs and abilities of the participants. Experiment, be creative, and find a flow that is right for you and your practitioners.

HOW THIS BOOK IS STRUCTURED

The book begins with warming up the joints and large muscle groups with the wheel (chapter 1). To minimize the risk of injury, it is advisable to warm up before each training session.

The following chapters are divided into different poses: Standing Poses, Arm Balance, Activation of the Core, Backbends, Forward Bends and Hip Openers, and Reverse Poses. The aim is to move from standing to the support and seated elements.

HOW THE EXERCISES ARE STRUCTURED

In addition to the explanatory text for each exercise, there is a brief list of which muscles are being used—that is, muscles that are stretched, activated, or strengthened. To perform the exercise correctly, it is recommended that you read the explanation in full before performing it. During the exercise, you should listen to your body's signals. The example on the following page shows how the poses are structured.

The exercises should only be performed if there is no pain and if no pain arises. When using the Yoga Wheel for the first time, a slow approach is recommended so as not to overstrain the body.

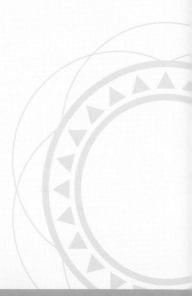

Name of the asana.

Photos of the different exercise variations.

List of the areas that will be strengthened, stretched or activated.

Detailed exercise description and description of how to breathe during the exercise.

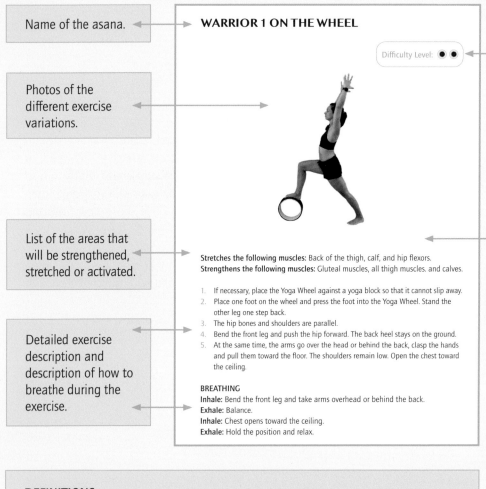

WARRIOR 1 ON THE WHEEL

Difficulty Level: ● ●

Stretches the following muscles: Back of the thigh, calf, and hip flexors.
Strengthens the following muscles: Gluteal muscles, all thigh muscles. and calves.

1. If necessary, place the Yoga Wheel against a yoga block so that it cannot slip away.
2. Place one foot on the wheel and press the foot into the Yoga Wheel. Stand the other leg one step back.
3. The hip bones and shoulders are parallel.
4. Bend the front leg and push the hip forward. The back heel stays on the ground.
5. At the same time, the arms go over the head or behind the back, clasp the hands and pull them toward the floor. The shoulders remain low. Open the chest toward the ceiling.

BREATHING
Inhale: Bend the front leg and take arms overhead or behind the back.
Exhale: Balance.
Inhale: Chest opens toward the ceiling.
Exhale: Hold the position and relax.

DEFINITIONS
Strengthens: Musculature is actively trained, strength increases, and muscle growth may occur.
Stretches: Musculature is pulled apart and stretched. Flexibility can improve.
Activates: Bring focus and concentration to the mentioned area.

HOW TO KNOW THE DIFFICULTY LEVEL

One circle: ●   Simple exercise

Two circles: ● ●   Challenging exercise (balance is needed)

Three circles: ● ● ●   Very difficult exercise (balance and strength are needed)

STARTING POSES

These typical starting poses will appear frequently in this book.

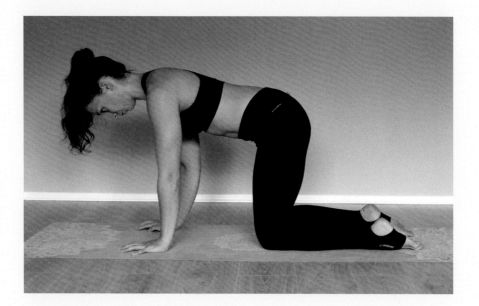

ALL FOURS

1. Place the knee joints under the hip bones.
2. The instep of the foot remains on the floor.
3. The wrists are below the shoulders.
4. The spine is in a neutral position by minimally tilting the pelvis forward and activating the building muscles.

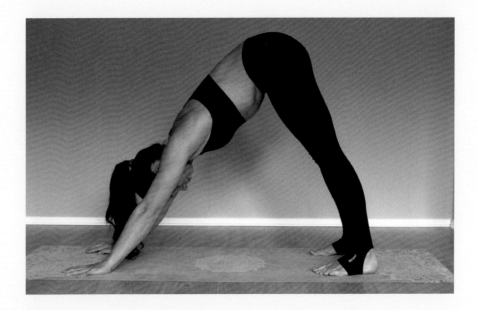

DOWNWARD DOG

1. From the All Fours, place the tips of your feet on the floor.
2. The hands are spread wide and pressed into the floor, the knee joints are stretched at the same time.
3. The heels actively pull into the floor.
4. The head and chest move between the arms and actively pull toward the thighs.
5. The pelvis remains tilted, the back long and straight.

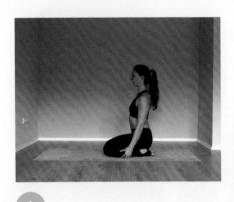

A

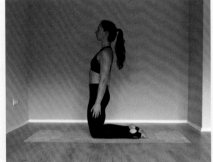

B

KNEELING SEAT AND KNEELING STAND

1. Start in a sitting position, bend the legs, place them on one side, and lift the buttocks.
2. The legs are closed.
3. Rest the buttocks on the heels for the kneeling position and raise the torso (photo *a*).
4. From the kneeling position, lift the buttocks off the heels until the hips are above the knee joints (photo *b*).
5. Keep the upper body upright and maintain tension in the abdominal muscles.

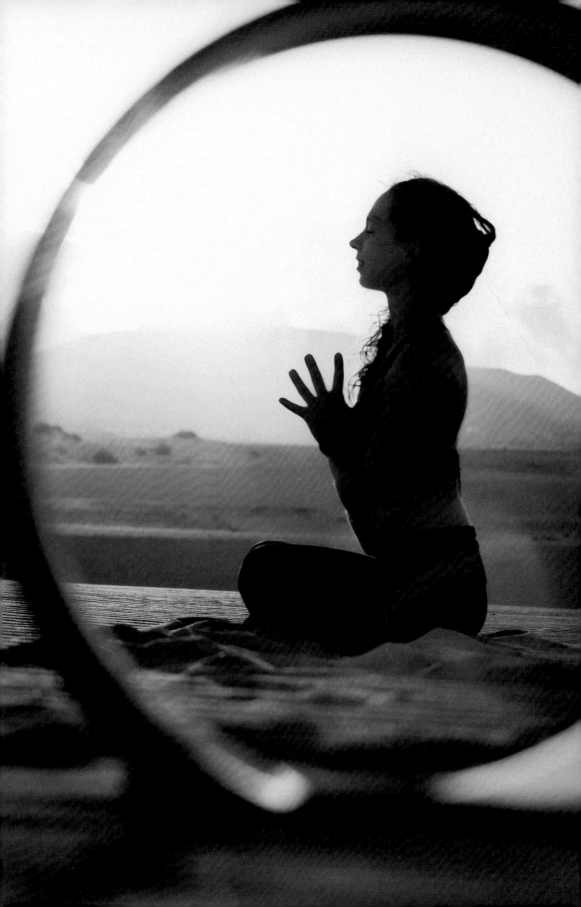

WARMING UP THE JOINTS AND LARGE MUSCLE GROUPS

THE WARM-UP

In society, yoga has to contend with the widespread prejudice of not being a strenuous sport and only serving as relaxation for older generations.

However, the opinion of yoga is increasingly in a state of change and gradually gaining recognition in Europe.

The versatility of yoga is reflected in the different styles, which differ in their execution. While classical Hatha Yoga is powerful, Vinyasa Yoga is characterized by its richness of sequences and a softer execution.

Although yoga styles differ significantly, they all generally start with a warm-up. Similar to soccer, swimming, or athletics, the warm-up plays a major role in yoga and can vary depending on the style. While one style tries to activate, tense as well as relax the muscles with the help of the breath and thoughts, another style mobilizes the most important joints.

There is no secret recipe for the perfect warming up and activation of the body, so the approach is up to the practitioner.

After many years of experience, I have found that mobilization and dynamic muscle activation is the best way to prepare my body for the Yoga Wheel sequences. The individual exercises with the Yoga Wheel are similar to the classic Sun Salutation and can be combined into a sequence.

The warm-up begins in a standing position. The legs, the largest muscle group in the body, are activated first. This is followed by the abdominal muscles. This is followed by mobilization and warming up of the spine and chest muscles.

The aim of the warm-up is to

- prepare the body for the yoga sequence, both mentally and physically,

- increase cardiac and respiratory performance,

- increase muscle blood circulation as well as muscle gliding ability,

- prevent injuries,

- produce joint fluid and thereby reduce joint stress, and

- create and improve motivation and increase concentration.

When practicing with the Yoga Wheel, it is strongly recommended to take 10–15 minutes to consciously warm up the individual body regions. This ensures a clean and concentrated execution.

SUN SALUTATION WITH THE YOGA WHEEL: MOUNTAIN POSE AND FORWARD BEND

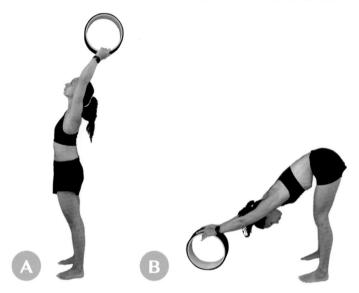

1. Start in a hip-width stance and bend the knees slightly for a stable stance.
2. Grasp the edge of the wheel and pull it over the head (photo *a*). Keep the elbows slightly bent.
3. Actively tense the gluteal muscles and open the chest. Pull the wheel slightly behind the head as a small counterweight.

BREATHING
Inhale: Open the chest.
Exhale: Put the wheel down in front.

4. Slowly release the position, and place the wheel on the floor, and move into a Forward Bend.
5. Place the palms of the hands on the wheel and pull the head between the arms (photo *b*).
6. Inhale and continue to move forward with the hands on the wheel, pulling the spine lengthwise.
7. Exhale and pull the shoulders back (away from the ears).

BREATHING
Inhale: Hands move forward.
Exhale: Pull the shoulders back.

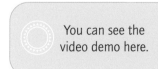
You can see the video demo here.

SQUAT WITH THE WHEEL

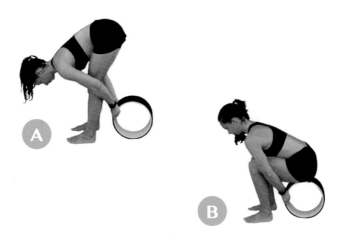

1. Staying in the Forward Bend, pull the wheel between the legs and place it behind the heels.
2. The hands go past the outside of the shin and try to grip the edge of the wheel (photo *a*).
3. Press the wheel into the floor and pull the upper body toward the wheel. Try to keep the back long and continue to open the torso.
4. Bend and straighten the knees for a squat with the wheel (photo *b*). Make sure that the knees are facing forward and remain behind the toes.

BREATHING
Inhale: Bend legs.
Exhale: Straighten legs.

MOUNTAIN CLIMBER ON THE WHEEL

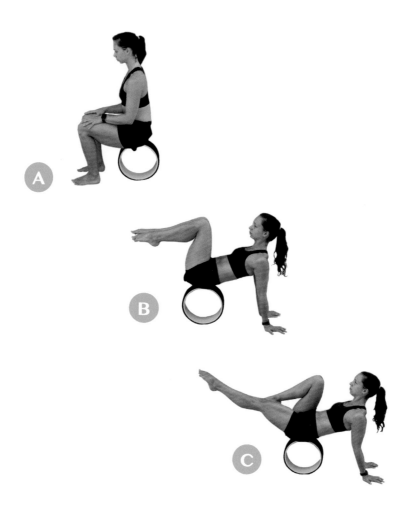

1. Remain seated completely on the wheel (photo *a*).
2. Place the hands shoulder width apart on the floor with all fingers pointing backward (photo *b*). If it is too wobbly, yoga blocks can be placed under the hands. The sacrum is now on the wheel. Try to lift both legs and balance.
3. When stable, alternately bend and stretch the legs to activate the abdominal muscles (photo *c*).

BREATHING
Breathe steadily throughout the execution of the exercise.

BACK INTO FORWARD BEND WITH WHEEL TRANSITION INTO ALL FOURS

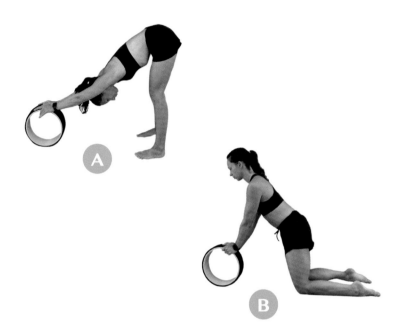

1. Place the feet back up and move back into a Forward Bend (photo *a*).

BREATHING
Inhale: Move back into a Forward Bend.

2. Bend both knee joints and place both on the floor to be in the All Fours position on the wheel (photo *b*).

BREATHING
Exhale: Place knees on the floor.

HAPPY CAT AND ANGRY CAT

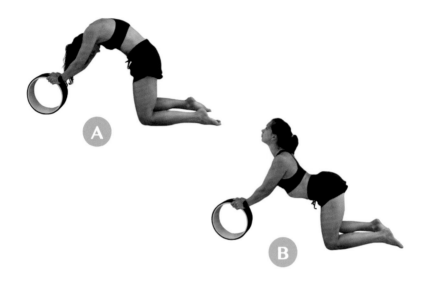

1. Press into the wheel with the hands and round the back for an Angry Cat (photo *a*).
2. Pull the chin to the chest as well.

BREATHING
Inhale: Round the back from cervical spine to lumbar spine.

3. Open the chest for a hollow back (Happy Cat; photo *b*).
4. Raise the head up.

BREATHING
Exhale: Relax the rounded position and bring the lower back into a slightly hollowed back.

COBRA AGAINST THE WHEEL

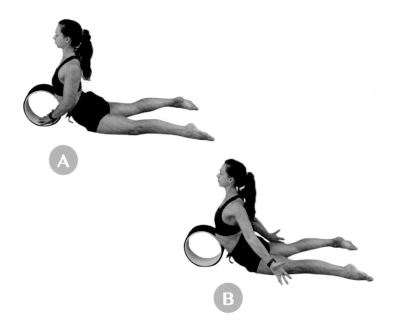

1. Slowly place the pubic bone on the floor and place the wheel on the sternum or abdominal wall. It is important that the pubic bone rests on the mat.
2. Place the hands on the inside of the wheel or stretch them out to the side to open the chest (photo *a*).
3. Tighten the gluteal muscles throughout the exercise and lower the shoulders as you exhale (photo *b*).

BREATHING
Inhale: Open the chest and pull the arms back.
Exhale: Lower the shoulders and open the chest more.

CHILD'S POSE ON WHEEL

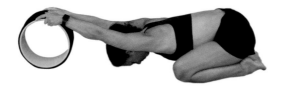

1. To briefly relieve the back, push the buttocks backward into a Child's Pose with the wheel.
2. Grasp the edge of the wheel and pull forward with the hands to lengthen the spine.

BREATHING
Inhale: Pull buttocks back toward heels.
Exhale: Hold briefly.
Inhale: Pull forward with hands.
Exhale: Pull shoulders back again.

FORWARD BEND AND MOUNTAIN POSE

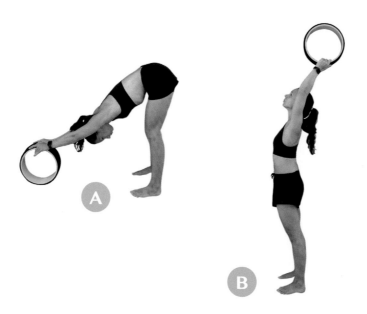

1. Coming out of child's pose, straighten the upper body and grasp the edge of the wheel.
2. From the upright child's pose, press the toes into the floor. Then come back onto the feet and run the feet under the hips (photo *a*).

BREATHING
Inhale: Straighten the upper body.
Exhale: Press the tips of the feet and heels into the floor while straightening the legs.
Inhale: Walk with feet forward.
Exhale: Hold in Forward Bend.

3. Continue to grasp the edge of the wheel and straighten the torso for a stretched Mountain Pose with the wheel.
4. Open the chest and move into a slight Backbend in the thoracic spine (photo *b*).

BREATHING
Inhale: Straighten the upper body and do a slight Backbend.
Exhale: Release tension and return to normal stance.

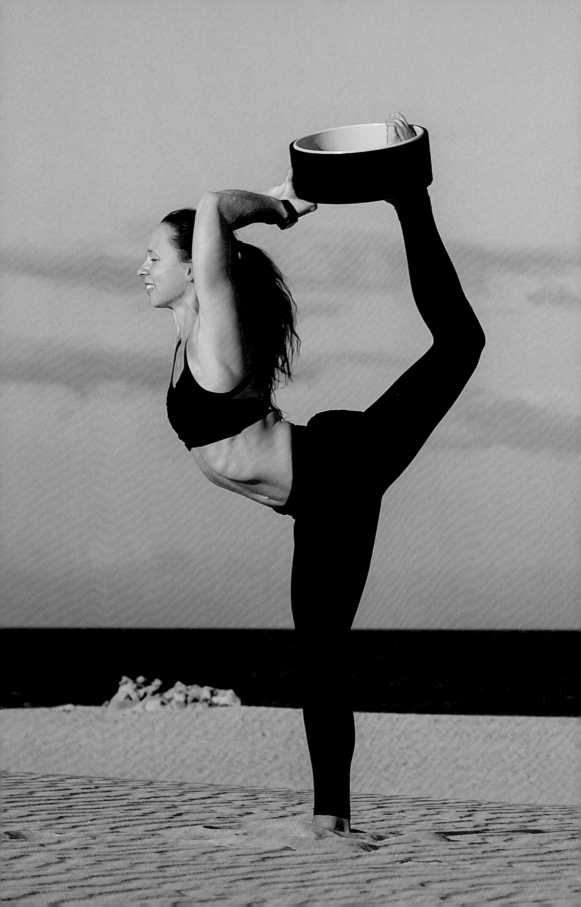

STANDING POSES

FORWARD BEND WITH LEGS NARROW AND WIDE APART

Difficulty Level: ◉

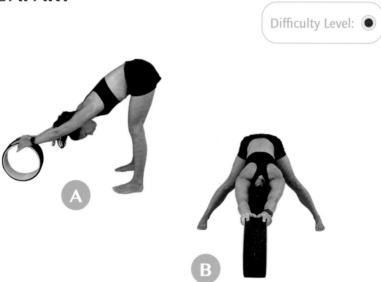

Stretches the following muscles: Back of thighs, inner thighs, calves, glutes, back extensors, and chest muscles.

1. Place the feet hip width (photo *a*) or further apart (photo *b*).
2. Place the wheel in the center and slowly roll forward with a straight back. Simultaneously tense abdominal and back muscles by pulling the belly button inward.
3. To increase the chest stretch, continue to roll forward slowly until the arms are fully extended.
4. The goal is to perform this exercise with a straight back and to bring the upper body toward the floor as far as possible.

BREATHING
Inhale: Place the hands on the wheel and keep the back long and straight.
Exhale: Hold the position and relax.

WIDE-LEG FORWARD BEND TWIST

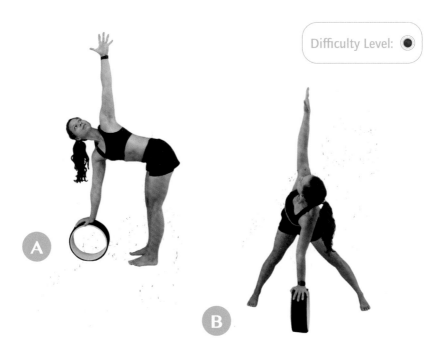

Difficulty Level: ◉

A

B

Stretches the following muscles: Back of the thighs, gluteal muscles, calves, pectoral muscles, and lateral trunk muscles.

1. Place the feet either hip width apart (photo *a*) or further apart (photo *b*).
2. Place the wheel in the center and roll it forward, keeping it aligned under the shoulders. Place one hand on top of the wheel.
3. Open the chest to the other side and tense the other arm to the ceiling. The gaze follows the arm.
4. If the wheel is too unstable, it can be fixed against a yoga block.

BREATHING
Inhale: The chest opens to the side.
Exhale: Hold the position and relax.

STRETCHED LATERAL ANGLE POSE

Difficulty Level: ●

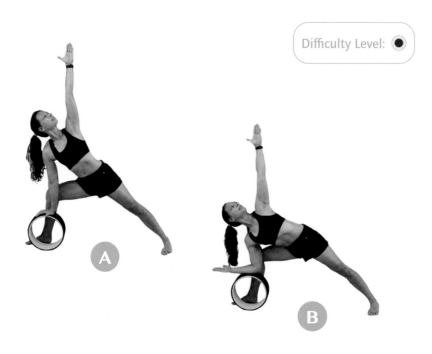

Stretches the following muscles: Inner thigh and back of the thigh, gluteal muscles, lateral trunk muscles, and pectoral muscles.

1. Start in a wide back lunge and turn the back foot at a 90-degree angle.
2. Bend the front leg, and make sure the knee joint is pointing in the same direction as the toe. The back leg is extended. Put the weight on the heel, outside of the foot.
3. Position the wheel next to the front foot and rest a hand on it. Balance the wheel. The other arm pulls toward the ceiling. The chest is opened forward (photo *a*).
4. If flexibility allows, the forearm can be placed on the wheel (photo *b*).

BREATHING
Inhale: Lunge, back foot at 90-degree angle.
Exhale: Place hand or forearm on wheel.
Inhale: Other arm pulls up toward the ceiling and opens the chest sideways.
Exhale: Hold the position and relax.

WARRIOR 1 ON THE WHEEL

Difficulty Level: ● ●

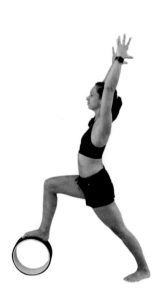

Stretches the following muscles: Back of the thigh, calf, and hip flexors.
Strengthens the following muscles: Gluteal muscles, all thigh muscles. and calves.

1. If necessary, place the Yoga Wheel against a yoga block so that it cannot slip away.
2. Place one foot on the wheel and press the foot into the Yoga Wheel. Stand the other leg one step back.
3. The hip bones and shoulders are parallel.
4. Bend the front leg and push the hip forward. The back heel stays on the ground.
5. At the same time, the arms go over the head or behind the back, clasp the hands and pull them toward the floor. The shoulders remain low. Open the chest toward the ceiling.

BREATHING
Inhale: Bend the front leg and take arms overhead or behind the back.
Exhale: Balance.
Inhale: Chest opens toward the ceiling.
Exhale: Hold the position and relax.

WARRIOR 2 ON THE WHEEL

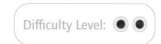

Difficulty Level: ● ●

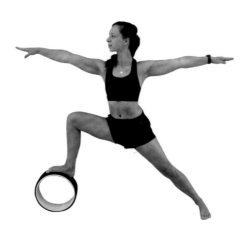

Stretches the following muscles: Inner thigh and hip flexors.
Strengthens the following muscles: Thigh muscles, gluteal muscles, and calves.

1. If necessary, place the Yoga Wheel against a yoga block so that it does not slip away.
2. Center one foot on the wheel and slide the other foot along the mat until the hips are open.
3. Place the back foot at a 90-degree angle and put weight on the heel and outside edge of the foot. Check that the back heel is aligned with the wheel.
4. The foot that is on the wheel remains fixed and actively pushes into the wheel. Bend the knee joint so that it is above the heel.
5. Raise arms to shoulder height and maintain the tension.

BREATHING
Inhale: Bend the front leg and raise the arms to shoulder height.
Exhale: Hold the position and relax.

WARRIOR 2 ON THE WHEEL VARIATIONS

Difficulty Level: ● ●

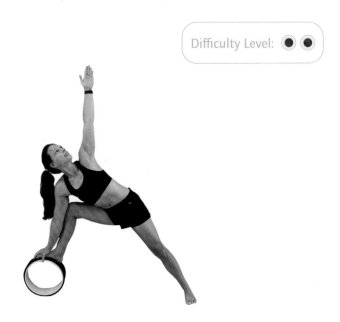

VARIATION 1

Stretches the following muscles: Inner thigh, hip flexors, lateral trunk muscles, and chest muscles.
Strengthens the following muscles: Gluteal muscles, thigh muscles, and calves.

1. From the Warrior 2 on the Wheel position, bring the front arm to the wheel, and rest the side of the body on the thigh.
2. The upper arm stretches up to the ceiling.

BREATHING
Inhale: Upper body leans forward; upper arm pulls toward the ceiling.
Exhale: Hold the position and relax.

Difficulty Level:

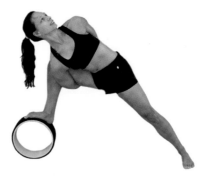

VARIATION 2

1. Release the hand from the wheel from variation 1 and bring it under the inner thigh.
2. Place the upper hand behind the back and grasp the lower hand. Open the chest forward.

BREATHING
Inhale: Bring the hands together behind the back.
Exhale: Hold the position and relax.

TRIANGLE POSE ON THE WHEEL

Difficulty Level: ● ●

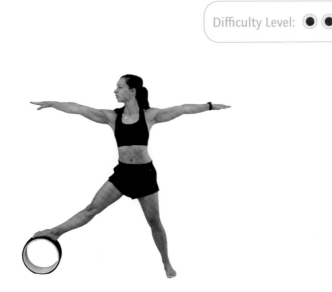

Stretches the following muscles: Inner thigh, hip flexors, lateral trunk muscles, and chest muscles.
Strengthens the following muscles: Gluteal muscles, thigh muscles, and calves.

1. From the Warrior 2 on the Wheel position, extend the leg that is on the wheel.
2. Extend the arms in line with the shoulders.
3. Bend the upper body sideways to the wheel. Pull one arm toward the floor, the other toward the ceiling.
4. The chest muscles open to the side.

BREATHING
Inhale: Extend the standing leg on the wheel and stretch the arms out to the side at shoulder height.
Exhale: Balance the position.
Inhale: The upper body bends sideways to the wheel; open the chest muscles to the side.
Exhale: Hold the position and relax.

SUN WARRIOR ON THE WHEEL

Difficulty Level: ● ●

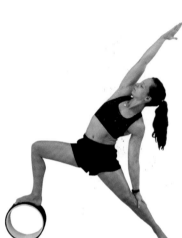

Stretches the following muscles: Inner thigh, hip flexors, and lateral trunk muscles.
Strengthens the following muscles: Gluteal muscles, hamstrings, and calves.

1. From the Warrior 2 on the Wheel position, bend the torso sideways to the back leg.
2. Support the rear hand on the calf so that the front arm can be actively pulled over the head and, at the same time, flex the trunk muscles to the side.

BREATHING
Inhale: Bend the trunk muscles sideways and pull the front arm over the head.
Exhale: Hold the position and relax.

LUNGE ON THE WHEEL

Difficulty Level: ● ● ●

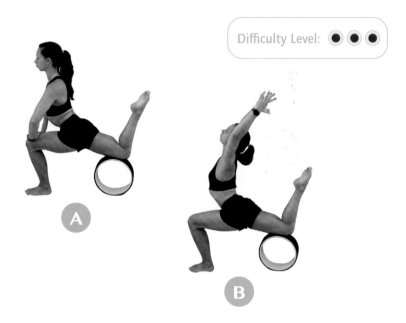

Stretches the following muscles: Front of the thigh and hip flexors.
Strengthens the following muscles: Gluteal muscles, hamstrings, and calves.

1. Start in a Downward Dog and place the wheel level with the knees.
2. Bring one leg between the hands and bend it, moving into a lunge.
3. Place the extended back leg above the knee (the knee joint should be free to move) on the wheel (photo *a*).
4. The hip remains parallel.
5. Actively press into the ground with the front leg and slowly straighten the upper body. The knee joint remains behind the toe.
6. Lift the hands off the floor and position either on the bent leg or sideways next to or above the head (photo *b*).

BREATHING
Inhale: From the Downward Dog looking down, step into a lunge.
Exhale: Place the back leg on the wheel.
Inhale: Actively press into the ground with the front leg and straighten the upper body.
Exhale: Hold the position and relax.

LUNGE ON THE WHEEL VARIATION

Difficulty Level: ● ● ●

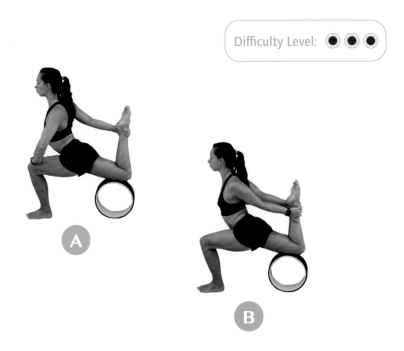

Stretches the following muscles: Front of the thigh and hip flexors.
Strengthens the following muscles: Gluteal muscles, hamstrings, and calves.

1. From the Lunge on the Wheel, bend and grasp the back leg by grabbing the foot with one hand (photo *a*).
2. Next, moving the other arm out to the side, grasp that same foot (photo *b*).
3. If you already have good flexibility in your back and hip flexors, you can grasp the foot using a Backbend in the spine.

BREATHING
Inhale: Bring the hand/hands to the foot and pull the leg close.
Exhale: Hold the position and relax.

STANDING ON THE WHEEL

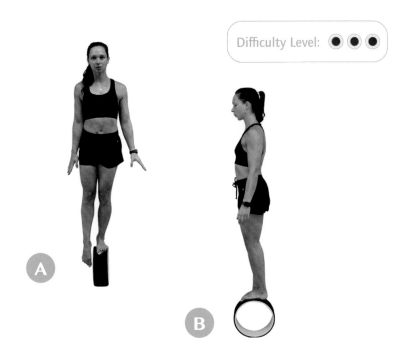

Difficulty Level: ● ● ●

A

B

Activates the following muscle areas: Sense of balance, arch of the foot, thigh, and trunk muscles.

1. Fix the wheel between two yoga blocks if needed.
2. Place the right foot next to the Yoga Wheel. Then step on the top of the wheel with the left foot (photo *a*). In the beginning, the wall can be used as a support.
3. Bend the knee of the standing leg slightly (photo *b*) and bring the hips into a parallel position.
4. Keep the free leg in the air at hip level and balance.
5. To make the exercise more difficult, remove the back block or both blocks first.

BREATHING
Inhale: Get on the wheel and lift the back leg off the ground.
Exhale: Balance on the wheel.

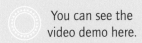 You can see the video demo here.

WARRIOR 3 ON THE WHEEL

Difficulty Level: ● ● ●

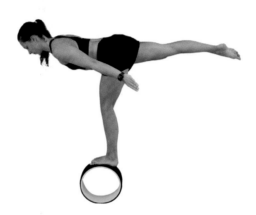

Strengthens the following muscles: Thigh muscles, gluteal muscles, trunk muscles, and arch of the foot.

1. Get into the Standing on the Wheel pose with yoga blocks.
2. Slowly lean forward with the upper body, and slowly stretch the free leg back until the leg is at the height of the upper body.
3. To begin and for support, the hands can hold on to the wall.
4. The standing leg remains slightly bent and the chest is open.

BREATHING
Inhale: Slowly lean forward with the upper body.
Exhale: Extend the leg backward.

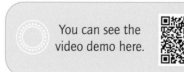

You can see the video demo here.

DANCER ON THE WHEEL

Difficulty Level: ● ● ●

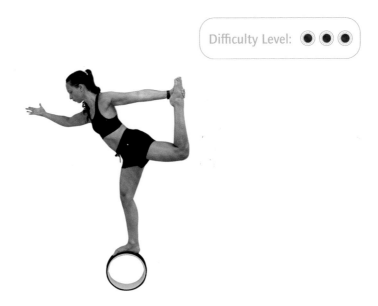

Strengthens the following muscles: Thigh muscles, gluteal muscles, arch of the foot, and lower back muscles.

Stretches the following muscles: Chest muscles, front shoulder, and abdominal muscles.

1. Get into the Standing on the Wheel pose with yoga blocks.
2. Bend the free leg and grasp the foot from the inside.
3. Slowly lean slightly forward with the upper body and press the foot into the hand. Slowly lift the leg a little.
4. To begin and for support, the hands can always hold on to the wall.
5. The standing leg remains slightly bent and the upper body is upright.

BREATHING

Inhale: Slowly lean the upper body forward and press into the hand and foot.

Exhale: Balance.

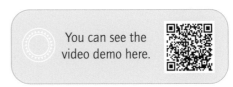

You can see the video demo here.

HAND-FOOT BALANCE FORWARD AND SIDEWAYS

Difficulty Level: ● ● ●

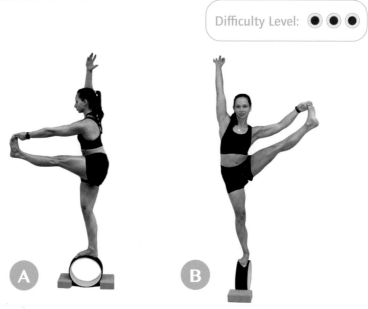

Strengthens the following muscles: Thigh muscles, gluteal muscles, arch of the foot, trunk muscles, and lower back muscles.

Stretches following muscles: Back of the thigh, inner thigh, calf muscles.

1. Get into the Standing on the Wheel pose with yoga blocks.
2. Bend the free leg and grasp the foot at the front of the big toe.
3. Try to stretch it slowly forward (easier version; photo *a*) or to the side (harder version; photo *b*).
4. To begin and for support, the hands can rest against the wall.
5. The standing leg remains slightly bent and the upper body is upright.

BREATHING

Inhale: Grasp toe and extend leg forward or to the side.

Exhale: Balance.

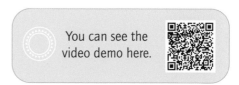

You can see the video demo here.

FORWARD AND SIDE PISTOL SQUAT ON THE WHEEL

Difficulty Level: ● ● ●

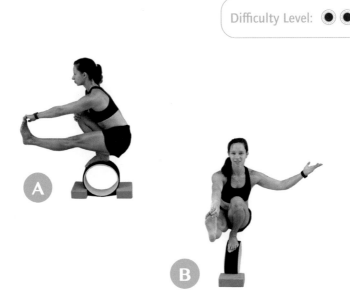

Strengthens the following muscles: Thigh muscles, gluteal muscles, hip flexor, and calf muscles.
Stretches the following muscles: Back of the thigh and calf muscles.

1. Get into the Standing on the Wheel pose with yoga blocks.
2. Bend the standing leg and slowly lower the buttocks toward the floor.
3. Raise the arms above the head. The upper body remains upright during the pose.
4. Grab the big toe of the extended leg and pull it forward (side view: photo *a*; front view: photo *b*) or to the side (hip opening).
5. When opening to the side, make sure to active the lateral abdominal muscles as well.

BREATHING
Inhale: Bend standing leg and lower buttocks.
Exhale: Grasp big toe and pull leg up.

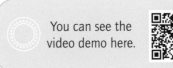
You can see the video demo here.

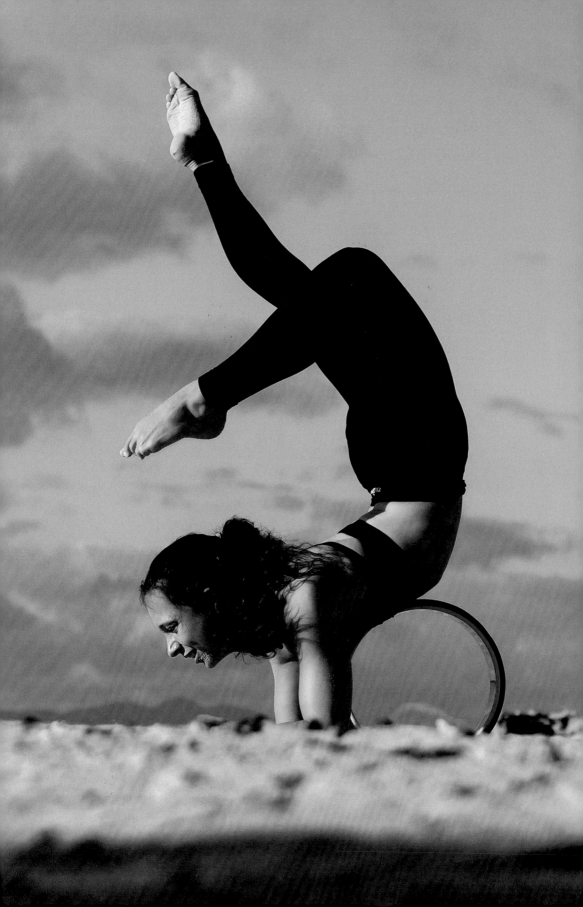

3

ARM
BALANCE

SHOULDER STAND

Difficulty Level: ● ●

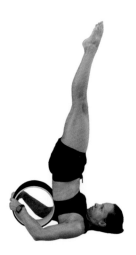

Strengthens the following muscles: Back muscles as well as abdominal muscles.
Activates the following muscles: Gluteal and leg muscles.

1. Start in the sitting position and place the wheel at lower back level. Roll completely over the wheel and rest head and shoulders on the floor. Lift the legs and pull them toward the face first.
2. Grasp the wheel with the hands and actively press it against the upper back.
3. Slowly lift the buttocks first and bring the back into a straight position. Tighten the abdomen and slowly push the legs up until they are extended.
4. If the back muscles are not yet strong enough, lift the legs only so far that the lower back is straight.
5. Dynamic variations:
    a. Dynamic movement: Pull the legs back toward the chest and actively push them back up toward the ceiling.
    b. Dynamic movement: Open the legs into a straddle, bring them to the floor, and slowly close them again.

BREATHING
Regular breathing throughout the exercise.

PUSH-UP ON THE WHEEL

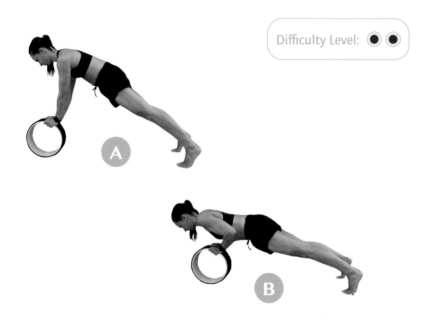

Difficulty Level: ● ●

Strengthens the following muscles: Chest muscles, posterior upper arm muscles, anterior shoulder muscles, abdominals, back muscles, and gluteal muscles.

1. Start in a kneeling position and place the wheel in front of the knees. Using the hands, walk the wheel forward so that the body is in a diagonal line.
2. The hands grip the edge of the wheel and press it into the floor.
3. The knees remain on the floor or are extended through so that the weight is only on the hands and the toes (photo *a*).
4. The pelvis tilts forward to activate the abdominal muscles and lock the lower back. Maintain this position throughout the exercise.
5. Start in the extended arm position and bend the elbows slowly, in a controlled manner, close to the body (photo *b*).
6. Actively push into the wheel to straighten the arms again.

BREATHING
Inhale: Bend the arms.
Exhale: Straighten the arms.

FIREFLY PREP ON THE FLAT WHEEL

Difficulty Level: ● ● ●

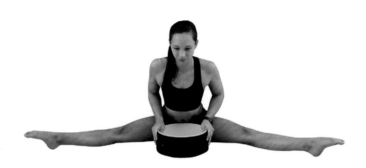

Strengthens the following muscles: Arm and shoulder muscles, all the back and abdominal muscles, and all the leg muscles.

1. Start in a straddle and place the wheel in between.
2. Lay the wheel on its side and place the hands either side of the wheel. The thumbs are on the inside and the remaining fingers are on the outside.
3. Bring the upper body to a 45-degree angle over the wheel. At the same time, bend the arms.
4. Tighten the entire abdomen and gluteal muscles.
5. Actively press into the wheel and lift the buttocks off the floor (see photo *a* for Firefly on the Flat Wheel on the following page). Stretch the arms to lift the remaining part of the legs off the floor.
6. Keep only the feet on the ground and press into the ground.
7. Repeat this exercise several times to prepare the chest and abdominal muscles for the Firefly on the Wheel.

BREATHING
Inhale: The upper body leans forward into the 45-degree angle and the arms bend.
Exhale: Press into the wheel and
straighten the arms.

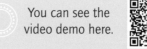
You can see the video demo here.

FIREFLY ON THE FLAT WHEEL

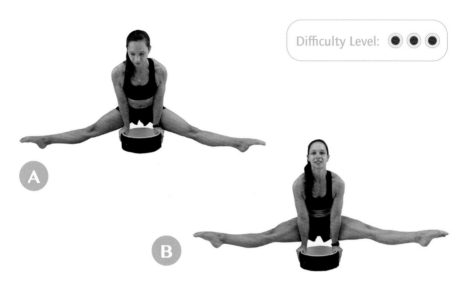

Difficulty Level: ● ● ●

Strengthens the following muscles: Arm and shoulder muscles, all the back and abdominal muscles, and all the leg muscles.

1. Start in a straddle and place the wheel on its side in front.
2. Place the hands on the side of the wheel (photo *a*). The thumbs are on the inside and the remaining fingers are on the outside.
3. Actively press into the floor with the hands, and activate the lower abdominal muscles as well as hip flexors and hamstrings to lift the legs off the floor (photo *b*).
4. Keep the legs slightly bent at the beginning to build balance and strength. The goal is to straighten the legs and open the chest.

BREATHING
Inhale: Place the hands on the wheel.
Exhale: Build strength and push into the wheel.
Inhale: Activate the abdominal muscles and lift the legs.
Exhale: Hold the position and relax.

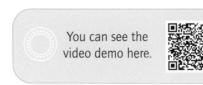

You can see the video demo here.

FIREFLY ON THE WHEEL

Difficulty Level: ● ● ●

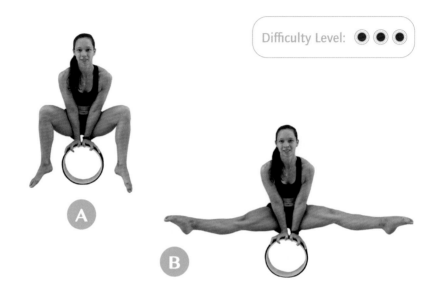

Strengthens the following muscles: Arm muscles, shoulder muscles, all back muscles, chest muscles, front of the thighs, and abdominal muscles.

1. Place the wheel with the opening toward the body, bend at the hips, and bring your legs a little farther apart so that the hands can reach the wheel.
2. Place the hands in the center on the wheel, with the thumb and index finger on the edge of the wheel. The other fingers are placed on the rubber coating.
3. Walk the feet forward slightly until they are bent sideways next to the wheel (photo *a*).
4. Build strength in the upper body and arms, and actively push into the wheel with the hands. The chest opens forward. Slowly lift the feet off the ground. Balance with the hands at the same time.
5. If the weight can be balanced on the wheel, there is an opportunity to stretch the legs (photo *b*). The back should remain straight.

BREATHING
Regular breathing throughout
the exercise.

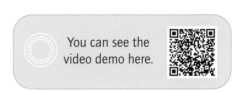

You can see the video demo here.

CROW

Difficulty Level:

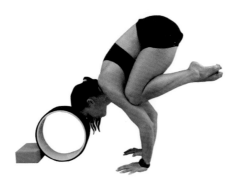

Strengthens the following muscles: Arm and shoulder muscles, as well as abdominal and lower back muscles.

1. Place the wheel half a step away against a yoga block.
2. Start in a squat position and place the hands shoulder width apart on the floor.
3. Place the knees to the side of the shoulder, or on the back of the upper arm.
4. Place the hairline of the forehead on the Yoga Wheel.
5. Actively squeeze the legs to activate the abdominal muscles and push the buttocks up. Try to release the legs from the floor alternately.
6. With sufficient balance, release both feet from the floor.
7. Shift the weight gradually to the hands.
8. Pull the buttocks up a little further by pulling the feet up.

BREATHING
Inhale: Lift the feet off the floor.
Exhale: Push the buttocks upwards.

CROW WITH FEET ON THE WHEEL

Difficulty Level: ● ● ●

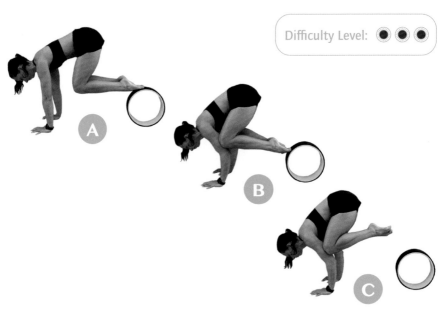

Strengthens the following muscles: Arm and shoulder muscles, as well as abdominal and lower back muscles.

1. Start in the Downward Dog position and place the top of each foot, one foot at a time, on the wheel. Apply pressure to the wheel at specific points.
2. Walk the hands forward a little to bring the body into a horizontal position. The hands are now under the shoulders (photo *a*).
3. Build abdominal tension and hold it throughout the exercise.
4. Actively press into the floor with the hands, simultaneously activating and opening the shoulders.
5. Pull the knees in toward the chest and bend the arms.
6. When sufficiently stable, open the legs shoulder width apart and rest the knees at shoulder or posterior upper arm level (photo *b*).
7. Squeeze the legs together gradually to activate the abdominal muscles and lift the buttocks slightly.
8. Try to slowly release the feet from the wheel and balance on the hands (photo *c*).

BREATHING
Inhale: Pull the legs close and bend the arms.
Exhale: Rest the knees on the back upper arm.
Inhale: Squeeze the legs together and release the feet from the wheel.
Exhale: Hold the position and balance.

CROW ON THE WHEEL

Difficulty Level: ● ● ●

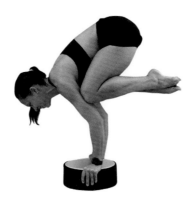

Activates and strengthens the following muscles: Arm and shoulder muscles, the whole back, and abdominal muscles.

1. Lay the wheel on its side and place the hands on the side of the wheel. The thumbs point inward. The remaining fingers are on the outside of the wheel and press inward.
2. Move into a slight squat and bend the arms.
3. Shift the weight forward and place the knees either:
    a. Laterally next to the shoulder (easier).
    b. Directly on the back part of the upper arm (more difficult).
3. Press the knees against each of the above points and inward at the same time to tighten the abdominal muscles.
4. Shift the weight forward and release first one, then both feet from the floor. Hold the tension.
5. If needed, alternate releasing the feet from the floor and slowly approach the feeling of body balance.

BREATHING
Inhale: Place the hands on the wheel and bring the knees into position.
Exhale: Build up strength. Push the legs inward and push into the wheel at the same time.
Inhale: Lift one or both feet off the floor.

CROW WITH ONE HAND ON THE WHEEL

Difficulty Level:

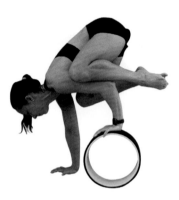

Activates and strengthens the following muscles: Arm and shoulder muscles, the whole back, and abdominal muscles.

1. Fix the wheel to a yoga block at the beginning.
2. Place one hand on the wheel and the other on the floor at the level of the yoga block. Bend the arm that is on the Yoga Wheel; the other arm remains stretched.
3. Place the same knee as the bent arm on the upper arm.
4. Apply pressure on both hands by activating the shoulder and abdominal muscles.
5. Push the buttocks more toward the ceiling, slowly release the foot from the floor, and pull it toward the buttocks.
6. Increase in difficulty: Perform the exercise without the yoga block.

BREATHING
Inhale: Place one hand on the wheel and the other on the floor.
Exhale: Place the knee on the arm that is on the wheel.
Inhale: Raise the buttocks to the ceiling and release the foot from the floor.
Exhale: Hold the position and relax.

HANDSTAND STRADDLE

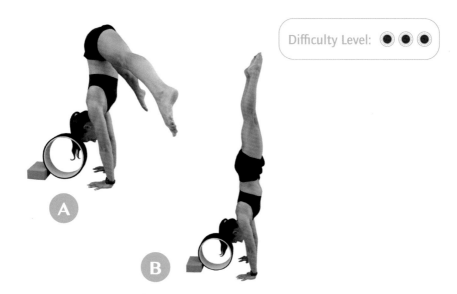

Difficulty Level: ● ● ●

Strengthens the following muscles: Hand, arm, and shoulder muscles as well as abdominal and lower back muscles.

1. Fix the wheel against a yoga block or a wall.
2. Start half a step away from the wheel in a hip-width stance and bend the upper body forward. Place the hands shoulder width apart on the floor. At the same time, rest the top of the head (not the forehead but the hairline!) on the wheel.
3. Bring the legs into a wide straddle and actively push the buttocks up so that they are almost above the head. Put weight on the wheel with the head.
4. Activate the abdominal and back muscles. First release one leg from the floor. At the same time, actively press the hands into the floor and activate the shoulders. If mobility is lacking in the legs, the feet can be placed on two additional yoga blocks to allow the buttocks to move over the head.
5. If strength and balance allow, release the other leg and move into a straddle (photo *a*). Push the buttocks farther toward the ceiling and bring the back into a straight position (no hollow back!).
6. With sufficient stability on the hands and strength in the center of the body, the legs can be brought together from the straddle, over the sides to the top into a handstand (photo *b*).

BREATHING
Inhale: Slowly lift the legs off the floor.
Exhale: Push out from the shoulders.

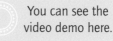 You can see the video demo here.

CHESTSTAND ON THE WHEEL I

Difficulty Level: ● ● ●

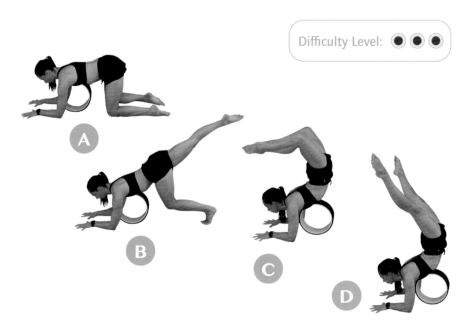

Strengthens the following muscles: All back muscles, shoulder muscles, forearm muscles, and gluteal muscles.

1. Start on all fours with forearms on the floor and place the wheel on the sternum and upper abdomen (photo *a*).
2. Keep the shoulder stable by actively pressing the forearms into the floor.
3. Come up on the toes and kick one leg up several times at first (photo *b*).
4. To maintain the Chest Stand, actively tighten the glutes and pull the legs overhead (photo *c*). Face the front.
5. If the sternum or upper abdomen lifts off the wheel, try to shift the weight back.
6. If there is enough strength in the lower back and glutes, the legs can also be stretched (photo *d*).
7. Throughout the exercise, the forearms actively press into the floor. Maintain tension in the glutes.

BREATHING
Inhale: Kick one leg up.
Exhale: Balance and try to pull the second leg up with it.
Inhale: Pull the legs over the head.
Exhale: Balance or stretch them.

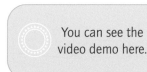 You can see the video demo here.

ELBOW LEVER ON THE WHEEL

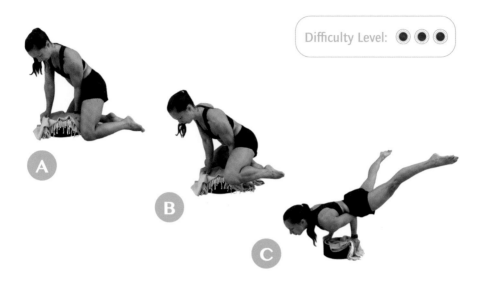

Difficulty Level: ● ● ●

Strengthens the following muscles: Shoulder girdle, arm muscles, chest muscles, abdominal muscles, glutes, and muscles of the legs.

1. Place the wheel on the side and start in a kneeling position.
2. Use a towel or blanket to pad the hard edge of the wheel and place the hands as follows (a clock helps as a guide): right hand at 1:00, left hand at 7:00 (photo *a*). The other way around would be with the left hand at 11:00 and right hand at 5:00.
3. Raise the buttocks from a kneeling position and round the lower back, engaging the abdominal muscles to create tension (photo *b*).
4. Bend the lower elbow and place it next to the pelvic bone. Put some weight on the elbow.
5. Keeping the front arm extended, press into the wheel and try to keep the knees bent off the ground.
6. When the legs can be kept in the air, the front arm can be slowly bent outward and the upper body can lean forward. The chest will still remain open.
7. Tighten the gluteal muscles and try to stretch the legs backward and upward (photo *c*).

BREATHING
Inhale: Lift knees off the floor.
Exhale: Slowly lean the upper body forward.

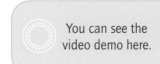
You can see the video demo here.

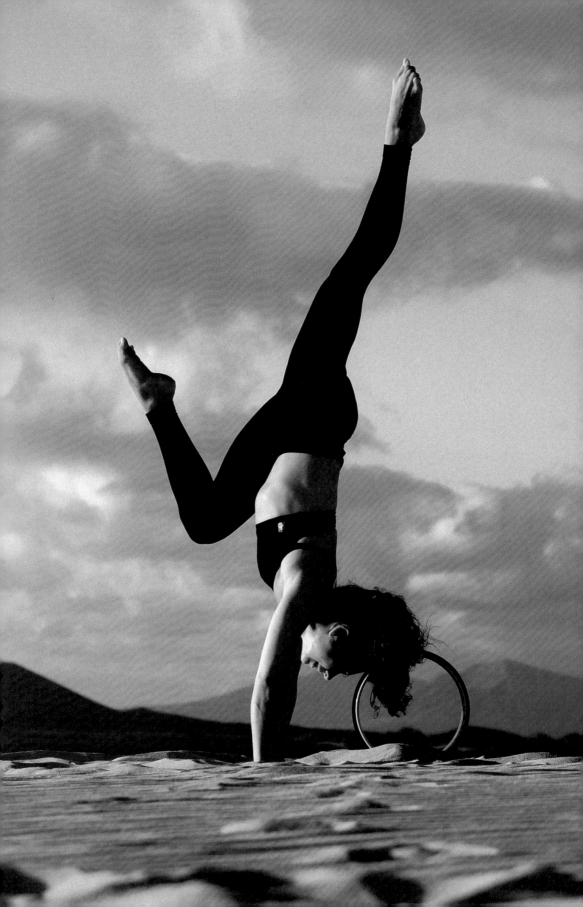

ACTIVATING
THE CORE

PLANK ON THE WHEEL

Difficulty Level:

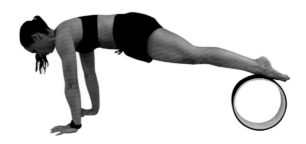

Strengthens the following muscles: Straight abdominal muscles, lower back muscles, upper back muscles, chest muscles, and arm muscles.

1. Start in a Downward Dog position and place one foot instep at a time on the wheel. Apply pressure to the wheel.
2. Move the hands forward to position them under the shoulders and bring the body into a horizontal position.
3. Tilt the pelvis forward so that the lower back rounds slightly and the abdominal muscles are tight (no hollow back!).
4. Pull the ribs inward and hold the tension.
5. Actively press into the floor with the hands, at the same time activating and opening the shoulders.
6. Hold the exercise for 30 seconds, pause, and then hold again.

BREATHING
Regular breathing throughout the exercise.

ONE-LEG PLANK ON THE WHEEL

Difficulty Level: ◉

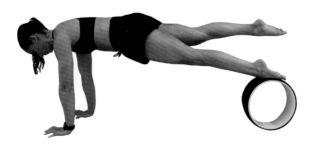

Strengthens the following muscles: Straight abdominal muscles, lower back muscles, upper back muscles, chest muscles, and arm muscles.

1. Starting pose: Plank on the Wheel.
2. Tilt the pelvis forward so that the lower back rounds slightly and the abdominal muscles are tense (no hollow back!).
3. Pull the ribs inward and hold the tension.
4. Actively press into the floor with the spread hands, simultaneously activating and opening the shoulders.
5. Alternately lift one leg and place it back on the wheel. The pressure on the wheel remains constant.

BREATHING
Inhale: Lift one leg.
Exhale: Put the leg down again.

DYNAMIC PLANK ON THE WHEEL

Difficulty Level: ● ●

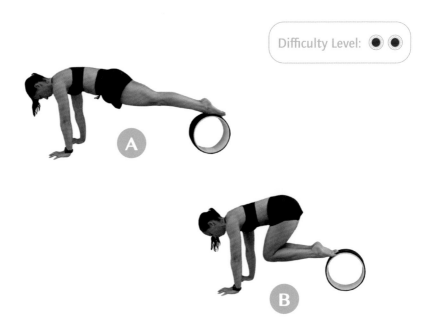

Strengthens the following muscles: Straight abdominal muscles, lower back muscles, upper back muscles, chest muscles, and arm muscles.

1. Starting pose: Plank on the Wheel.
2. Tilt the pelvis forward so that the lower back rounds slightly (photo *a*) and the abdominal muscles are tense (no hollow back!).
3. Pull the ribs inward and hold the tension.
4. Actively press into the floor with the spread hands, simultaneously activating and opening the shoulders.
5. Pull the knees toward the chest, thereby rolling the wheel back and forth (photo *b*). The rolling direction should always be straight.
6. The movements take place exclusively in the legs. The upper body holds the tension. Keep the entire back in a straight line.

BREATHING
Inhale: Draw the knees in toward the chest.
Exhale: Straighten the knees again and lengthen the body.

RIGHT-ANGLE PLANK

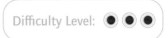

Difficulty Level: ● ● ●

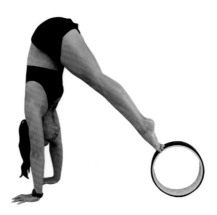

Strengthens the following muscles: Straight abdominal muscles, lower back muscles, upper back muscles, chest muscles, and arm muscles.

1. Starting pose: Plank on the Wheel.
2. Tilt the pelvis forward so that the lower back is slightly rounded and the abdominal muscles are tense (no hollow back!).
3. Pull the ribs inward and hold the tension.
4. Actively press into the floor with the spread hands, simultaneously activating and opening the shoulders.
5. Slowly lift the buttocks toward the ceiling. Meanwhile, minimally pull the wheel to the center of the body.
6. Final position, and therefore the full amplitude of movement, is when the buttocks are above the head. The body forms a right angle at the hips.
7. Hold the tension and bring the buttocks back down to a horizontal position with the same tension.

BREATHING
Inhale: Pull the buttocks toward the ceiling.
Exhale: Return the buttocks to a horizontal position.

SINGLE-LEG RIGHT ANGLE PLANK

Difficulty Level: ● ● ●

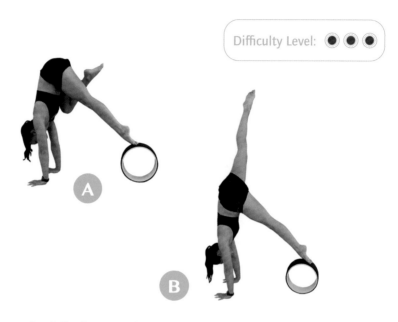

Strengthens the following muscles: Straight and oblique abdominal muscles, lower back muscles, upper back muscles, chest muscles, arm muscles.

1. Starting pose: Plank on the Wheel.
2. Tilt the pelvis forward so that the lower back rounds slightly and the abdominal muscles are tense (no hollow back!).
3. Pull the ribs inward and hold the tension.
4. Actively press into the floor with the spread hands, simultaneously activating and opening the shoulders.
5. Release one foot from the wheel and slowly push the buttocks toward the ceiling. The free leg can remain bent (easy variation; photo *a*) or stretched (advanced variation; photo *b*).
6. Final position, and therefore full amplitude of movement, is when the buttocks are overhead.
7. Hold the tension and bring the buttocks back down to horizontal with the same tension.
8. Change the instep.

BREATHING
Inhale: Pull the buttocks toward the ceiling.
Exhale: Return the buttocks to a horizontal position.

HANDSTAND TUCK

Difficulty Level: ● ● ●

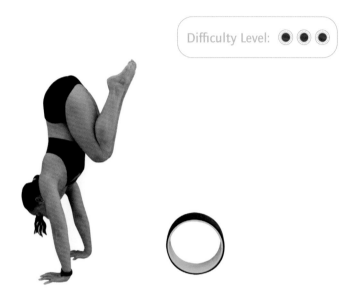

Strengthens the following muscles: Straight abdominal muscles, lower back muscles, upper back muscles, chest muscles, and arm muscles.

1. Starting pose: Plank on the Wheel.
2. Tilt the pelvis forward so that the lower back rounds slightly and the abdominal muscles are tense (no hollow back!).
3. Pull the ribs inward and hold the tension.
4. Actively press into the floor with the spread hands, at the same time activating and opening the shoulders.
5. Slowly lift buttocks and bring them over head. Balance at a right angle.
6. Bend one leg and bring it toward the chest.
7. Balance with the help of hands and release the other foot from the wheel, bend the leg and pull it toward the chest.
8. Hold the pose.
9. Variation: Bring the legs out of the pose and into a straddle.

BREATHING
Inhale: The buttocks pull toward the ceiling.
Exhale: Find and maintain balance.
Inhale: Release the feet one by one from the wheel.
Exhale: Balance.

HALF HEADSTAND

Difficulty Level: ● ●

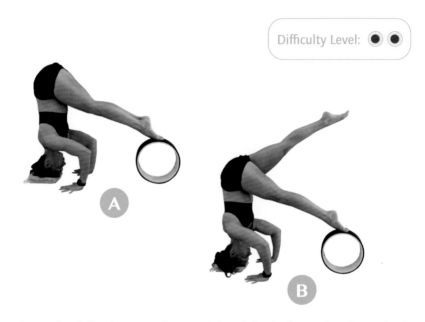

Strengthens the following muscles: Straight abdominal muscles, lower back muscles, upper back muscles, and arm muscles.

1. Start in All Fours and place the head on the floor. The wheel is between the legs.
2. Reposition the hands so that they are shoulder width apart and the elbows are in line with the wrists.
3. Place the top of the feet on the wheel and push the buttocks over the head (photo *a*).
4. At the same time, the hands press into the floor, and the shoulder muscles pull toward the buttocks.
5. Roll the wheel back and forth.
6. Variation: Hold in the Headstand pose and alternately lift one leg (photo *b*).

BREATHING
Inhale: Place the head on the floor.
Exhale: Place the feet on the wheel.
Inhale: The buttocks push overhead.
Exhale: The buttocks push back.

VARIATION:
Inhale: Lift the leg.
Exhale: Change leg.

LATERAL BEND ON THE WHEEL

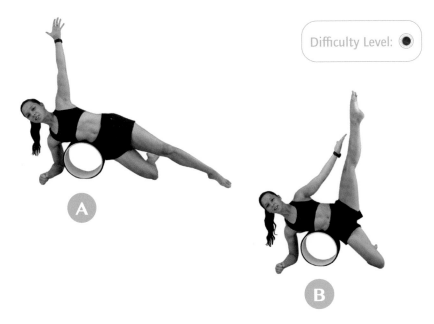

Difficulty Level: ●

Strengthens the following muscles: Lateral abdominal muscles, shoulder muscles, and the entire back muscles.

1. Start in a kneeling position. The wheel is sideways, next to the buttocks.
2. Place the lateral abdominal on the wheel. The lower arm is placed in line with the shoulder on the mat.
3. Roll a little higher until the buttocks are no longer in contact with the heels.
4. The inner leg remains bent, the outer leg stretches and stabilizes with the help of the foot (photo *a*).
5. Lift the upper leg slightly off the mat and balance (photo *b*). The weight shifts to the arm lying on the mat.

BREATHING
Inhale: Lie sideways on the wheel.
Exhale: Balance.
Inhale: Lift the leg off the mat.
Exhale: Hold the position and balance.

LATERAL BEND ON THE WHEEL VARIATIONS

Difficulty Level: ● ●

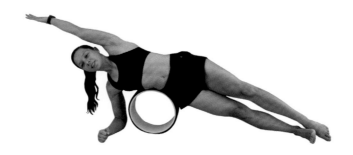

VARIATION 1

Strengthens the following muscles: Lateral abdominal muscles, shoulder muscles, and the entire back muscles.

1. Stretch the inner bent leg.

BREATHING
Regular breathing throughout the exercise.

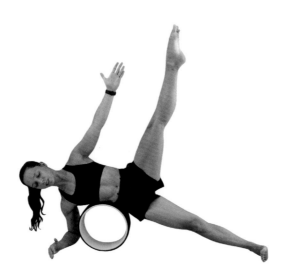

VARIATION 2

1. Start with either the inner bent leg or extended leg on the floor.
2. Dynamically bring the outer leg and arm alternately to the floor and ceiling.

BREATHING
Inhale: Take position.
Exhale: Balance.
Inhale: Bring the leg and arm to the ceiling.
Exhale: Return the leg and arm to the floor.

ABDOMINAL EXERCISE ON THE WHEEL I

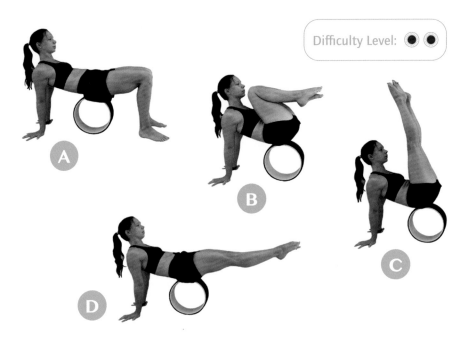

Difficulty Level: ● ●

Strengthens the following muscles: Entire abdominal muscles, lower back muscles, and shoulder and arm muscles.

1. Place the buttocks on the center of the wheel.
2. Place the arms at the sides of the wheel and walk back a little with the hands so that they are in a shoulder-lengthening position (photo *a*).
3. The hands are spread wide and point outward. While doing the exercise, keep them under the shoulders.
4. Slowly release the legs from the floor and pull them toward the chest (photo *b*).
5. Find the balance in this position. Keep the head in line with the back. Pull the ribs inward and tilt the pelvis forward minimally to tighten the abdominal muscles.
6. Straighten the legs toward the ceiling (photo *c*) and then slowly bring them parallel the floor (photo *d*). Avoid falling into a hollow back while doing this. Go only as low with the legs as the back and balance allow.
7. At the same time, press the arms into the floor to maintain the back position.
8. Return the legs to the ceiling in an extended position.

BREATHING
Inhale: Place the buttocks on the wheel.
Exhale: Balance.
Inhale: Straighten the legs and bring them to the floor.
Exhale: Raise the legs again.

ABDOMINAL EXERCISE ON THE WHEEL II

Difficulty Level: ● ●

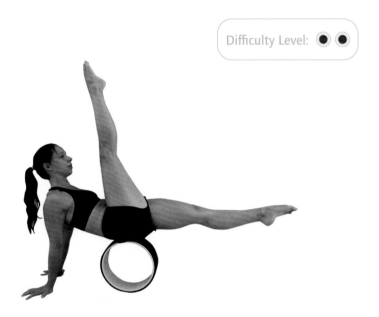

Strengthens the following muscles: Entire abdominal muscles, lower back muscles, and shoulder and arm muscles.
Activates the following area: Sense of balance.

1. Take the starting pose as in Abdominal Exercise on the Wheel I.
2. Alternately stretch the legs to the floor and ceiling.

BREATHING
Regular breathing during the exercise.

ABDOMINAL EXERCISE ON THE WHEEL III

Difficulty Level: ● ●

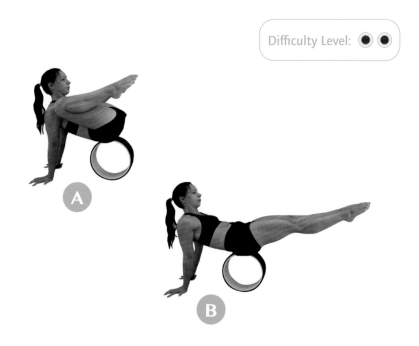

Strengthens the following muscles: Entire abdominal muscles, lower back muscles, and shoulder and arm muscles.

1. Start from the same position as in Abdominal Exercise on the Wheel I.
2. Bend both legs and bring the tips of the feet together. Open the knees to the side and pull toward the shoulders (photo *a*).
3. The knee joints are extended again, and the legs are brought forward (photo *b*).
4. Alternate bending and extending the knee joints. The tips of the feet remain together throughout the exercise.

BREATHING
Regular breathing during the exercise.

ABDOMINAL EXERCISE ON THE WHEEL IV

Difficulty Level: ● ●

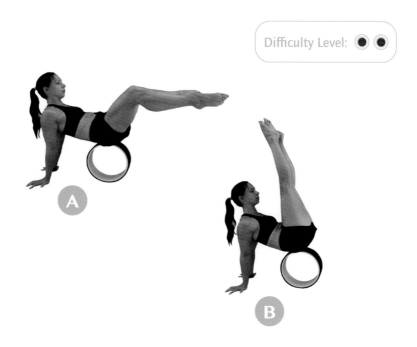

Strengthens the following muscles: Entire abdominal muscles, lower back muscles, shoulder, and arm muscles.

1. Start from the same position as in Abdominal Exercise on the Wheel I.
2. Stretch the legs and bring them close to the body.
3. Open the legs and bring them into a straddle (photo *a*). Then bring them back together in a semicircle in a horizontal position.
4. Then pull the stretched legs back toward the body (photo *b*).

BREATHING
Regular breathing during the exercise.

SIDE PLANK ON THE WHEEL I

Difficulty Level: ● ● ●

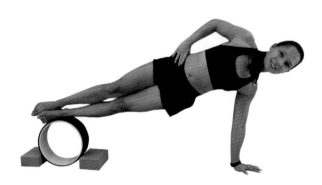

Strengthens the following muscles: Entire abdominal muscles, lower back muscles, and shoulder and arm muscles.

1. Start in a kneeling position, place the wheel sideways at hip level, and fix it with the yoga blocks.
2. From there, take the hand that is not on the side of the wheel and place it to the side under the shoulder.
3. Place the inner foot with the outer edge on the wheel, shift the weight on it, and slowly stretch the leg. Roll the wheel back a little more if necessary to help stretch the leg.
4. The upper leg can be placed as follows:
    a. In front of the body on the floor/another yoga block.
    b. On the inner thigh of the stretched leg.
    c. On the Yoga Wheel.
5. In all options, the hips are open forward and the body is in a line.
6. The exercise can be practiced either statically or dynamically by raising and lowering the pelvis sideways toward the ceiling.
7. Alternate between the two sides.

BREATHING
Regular breathing during the exercise.

SIDE PLANK ON THE WHEEL II

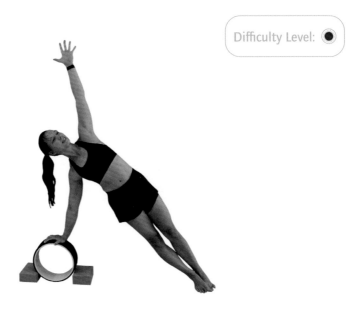

Difficulty Level: ⦿

Strengthens the following muscles: Entire abdominal muscles, lower back muscles, and shoulder and arm muscles.

1. Place the wheel against a yoga block to hold it in a fixed position.
2. Start in a kneeling position and place the inner part of the hand on the wheel.
3. Stretch both legs and place the inner foot with the outer edge on the floor. The outer foot is placed behind the inner one. Raise the hips at the same time.
4. Tense the entire core muscles and actively press the hand on the wheel into the ground.
5. The outer arm pulls up sideways.
6. The exercise can be practiced either statically or dynamically. The upper arm can be brought up alternately, close to the chest, to the floor, and to the ceiling.
7. Alternate between the two sides.

BREATHING
Regular breathing during the exercise.

SIDE PLANK ON THE WHEEL II VARIATIONS

Difficulty Level: ● ●

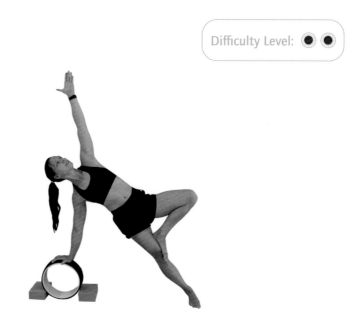

VARIATION 1

Strengthens the following muscles: Entire abdominal muscles, lower back muscles, and shoulder and arm muscles.

1. The starting pose is the Side Plank on the Wheel II.
2. Angle the outer leg and place the foot on the calf or thigh.
3. This exercise can be practiced either statically or dynamically by moving the pelvis up and down.

BREATHING
Regular breathing during the exercise.

Difficulty Level: ● ● ●

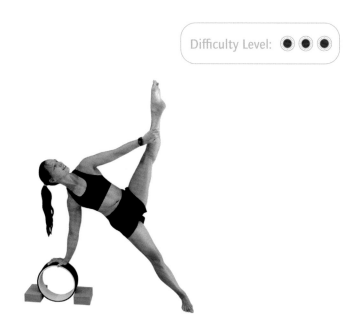

VARIATION 2

1. The starting pose is the Side Plank on the Wheel II.
2. Angle the outer leg and bring the outer hand to either the calf or heel.
   Try to straighten the leg.
3. Balance and pull the extended leg to the shoulder using the hand.

BREATHING
Regular breathing during the exercise.

INVERTED PLANK

Difficulty Level: ● ●

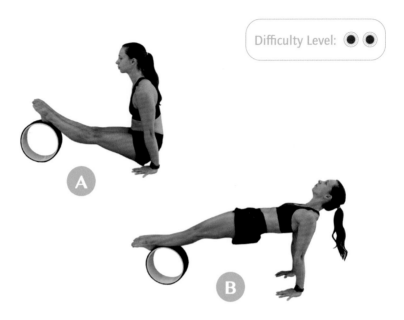

Strengthens the following muscles: Entire abdominal muscles, lower back muscles, and shoulder and arm muscles.
Stretches the following muscles: Front shoulder muscles, chest muscles, and upper arm muscles.

1. Start in a seated position and place the heels on the wheel.
2. Place the hands next to the buttocks with the fingertips pointing forward and stretch the legs (photo *a*).
3. Actively press into the floor and lift the buttocks off the floor.
    The chest is lifted to keep the torso straight.
4. The heels press into the wheel.
5. Push the hips up with the help of the wheel. Keep the abdominal, back, and gluteal muscles tense. The wheel is now under the calves (photo *b*).
6. Hold the tension and slowly roll back.
7. The exercise is performed dynamically.

BREATHING
Inhale: The hands press into the floor and the buttocks release.
Exhale: Push the hips up and bring the body into line.

SUMO SQUAT ON THE WHEEL

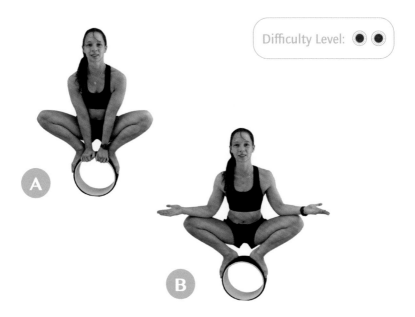

Difficulty Level: ● ●

Strengthens the following muscles: Entire abdominal muscles, lower back muscles, and leg muscles.
Stretches the following muscles: Inner thigh muscles.

1. Place the hands on the middle of the wheel. Grasp the front edge of the Yoga Wheel with the fingers.
2. Bend the legs and first place one foot on the wheel. The heels should be at the same level of the hands.
3. Shift the weight onto the wheel with the foot in a controlled manner and, at the same time, push with the other hand in the direction where of the other foot. This countermovement avoids falling over to the side.
4. Place the other foot on the wheel with the heel level with the hand (photo *a*).
5. Balance using the pelvis and the associated trunk muscles.
6. If balance is sufficient, the hands can be released from the wheel and placed on the legs (photo *b*) or raised above the head.
7. Easier alternative: place two yoga blocks next to the wheel to hold it in place. When balance is there, one yoga block can be released.

BREATHING
Regular breathing during the exercise.

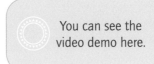 You can see the video demo here.

DYNAMIC SUMO SQUAT ON THE WHEEL

Difficulty Level: ● ● ●

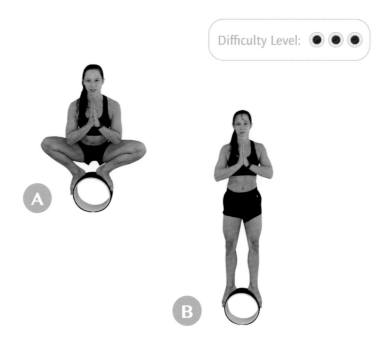

Strengthens the following muscles: Entire abdominal muscles, lower back muscles, and leg muscles.

1. Start in the Sumo Squat on the Wheel pose.
2. Bring the hands in front of the chest in a prayer position and press together tightly to engage the shoulder girdle and arm muscles to create tension (photo *a*).
3. Press the heels and the tops of the feet into the wheel and slowly try to straighten the knees.
4. Keep the upper body upright.
5. Try to extend the legs completely (photo *b*) and then bend them again and move back into the Sumo Squat.

BREATHING
Inhale: Push up and stretch the legs.
Exhale: Balance.
Inhale: Bend legs again and move back into the Sumo Squat.
Exhale: Balance in the Sumo Squat.

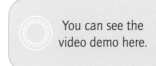
You can see the video demo here.

SITTING ON THE WHEEL (LONG SIDE)

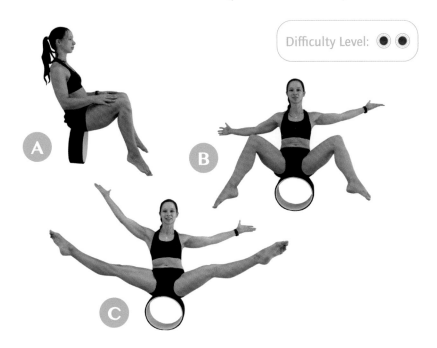

Difficulty Level: ● ●

Strengthens the following muscles: Entire abdominal muscles, lower back muscles, and leg muscles.

1. Place the sit bones on the front third of the Yoga Wheel.
2. Lean back slightly with the upper body and tense the abdominal muscles (photo *a*).
3. Slowly raise the legs and balance with the sit bones on the wheel.
4. The arms can be moved to balance (photo *b*).
5. Increase: Stretch the legs (photo *c*) and bend them again.

BREATHING
Regular breathing during the exercise.

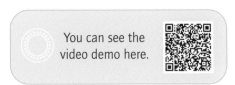

You can see the video demo here.

SITTING ON THE WHEEL (SHORT SIDE)

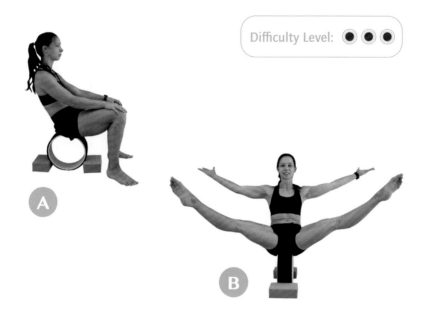

Difficulty Level: ● ● ●

A

B

Strengthens the following muscles: Entire abdominal muscles, lower back muscles, and leg muscles.

1.   Place the sacrum centrally on the wheel.
2.   Lean the upper body back a little and tense the abdominal muscles (photo *a*).
3.   Slowly lift the legs and balance with the sacrum on the wheel.
4.   The arms can be moved for balance.
5.   Increase: Stretch the legs (photo *b*) and bend them again.

BREATHING
Regular breathing during the exercise.

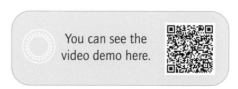

You can see the
video demo here.

SHIN BALANCE ON THE WHEEL

Difficulty Level: ● ●

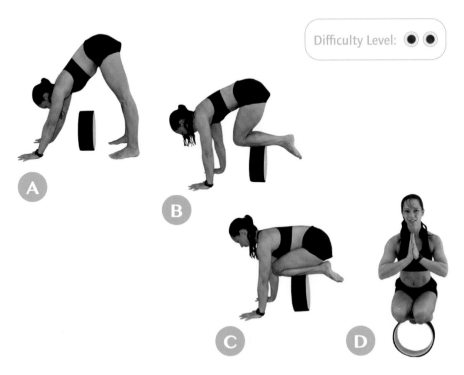

Strengthens the following muscles: Entire abdominal muscles, lower back muscles, and leg muscles.

1. Start in a Downward Dog and place the wheel under the chest (photo *a*).
2. Bend the knee joints and place the middle part of the shins on the wheel (photo *b*). Optionally, a blanket can be placed under the shins here.
3. Lower the buttocks toward the heels and try to open the chest again and let the back elongate (photo *c*).
4. Slowly release the hands from the floor and bring them together in a prayer position in front of the chest. Press the hands together to build tension in the upper body (photo *d*).
5. Easier variations:
   a. Fix the wheel with two yoga blocks.
   b. Use two yoga blocks straighten the upper body.

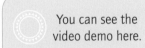
You can see the video demo here.

BREATHING
Regular breathing during the exercise.

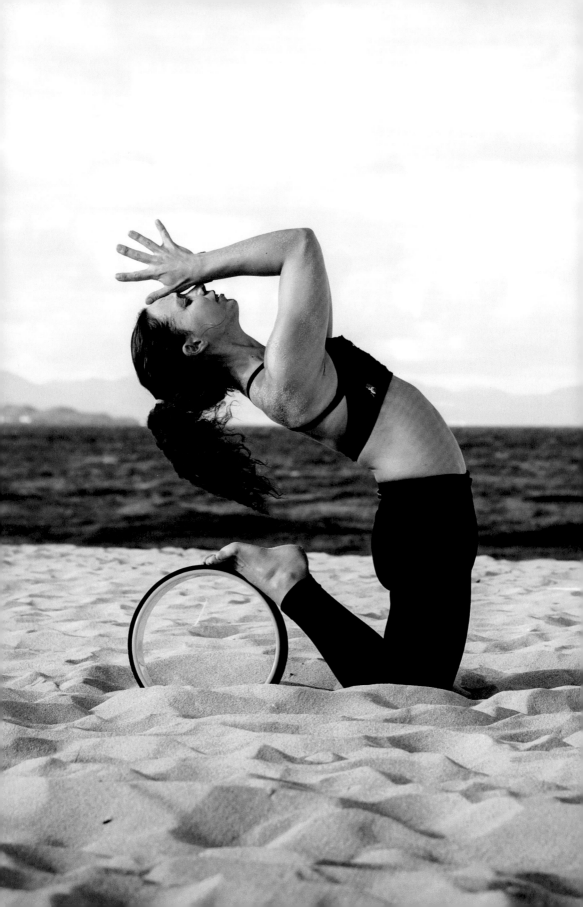

BACKBENDS

BACKBEND ON THE WHEEL

Difficulty Level: ◉ ◉

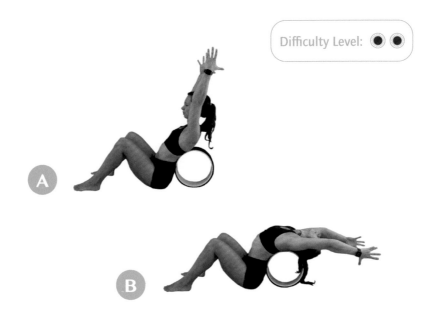

Stretches the following muscles: Abdominal and chest muscles and anterior shoulder muscles.

1. Rest the lower back on the wheel, and slowly lean back to rest the upper part of the back on the wheel.
2. Lift the arms above the head (photo *a*), pull the belly button inward, and rest the head on the wheel if sufficiently flexible (photo *b*).
3. The arms can remain above the head or be brought together at the back of the head.

BREATHING
Inhale: Place the upper part of the back on the wheel.
Exhale: Lift the arms above the head.
Inhale: Rest the head on the wheel.
Exhale: Hold the position and relax.

BACKBEND ON THE WHEEL VARIATIONS

Difficulty Level:

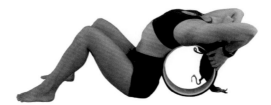

VARIATION 1

Stretches the following muscles: Abdominal and chest muscles and anterior shoulder muscles.

1. Bring the hands past the neck to grasp the wheel so that the shoulders and chest open wider.

BREATHING
Inhale: Move the hands past the neck and grasp the wheel.
Exhale: Hold the position and relax.

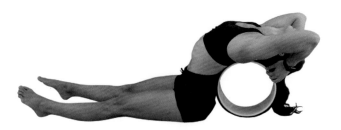

VARIATION 2

Stretches the following muscles: Abdominal and chest muscles and anterior shoulder muscles.

1. From variation 1, stretch the legs to further open the abdominal wall.

BREATHING
Inhale: Straighten the legs.
Exhale: Hold the position and relax.

BANANA ON THE YOGA WHEEL

Difficulty Level: ●

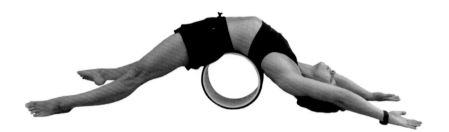

Stretches the following muscles: Abdominal muscles, chest muscle, and hip flexors.

1. From the Backbend on the Wheel pose, lift the buttocks a little, and place the lower back completely over the wheel. Roll over the wheel, and rest the head on the floor.
2. Pull the arms over the head and straighten the legs.
3. After a few breaths, bend the legs again, and roll further back to rest the head and shoulders.
4. Place the arms at the sides of the body, and stretch the legs, putting the feet on the floor. The knees can be bent so that there is not as much stretch in the hip flexors or abdominal wall.

BREATHING
Inhale: Lift the buttocks and rest the back on the wheel/rest head and shoulder on the floor.
Exhale: Stretch the arms over the head, open the chest.
Inhale: Straighten or bend the knees.
Exhale: Hold the position and relax.

PYRAMID ON THE WHEEL

Difficulty Level:

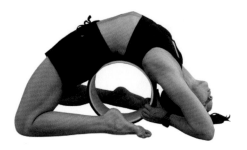

Stretches the following muscles: Abdominal muscles, chest muscles, hip flexors, and front of thigh.

1. Starting in a kneeling pose. Place the wheel above the tailbone.
    The hands are on the lower part of the wheel.
2. Activate the gluteal muscles and rest the lower back on the wheel.
    The hands move along the floor.
3. Pull the belly button in and rest the upper back on the wheel.
    Switch from the hands to the forearms.
4. When the whole back is completely on the wheel, maintain tension in
    the gluteal muscles. Take the arms above the head or, if flexible enough,
    grasp the wheel level with the neck.
5. In addition, the forearms can be lowered if the chest muscles allow it.

BREATHING
Inhale: Slowly lay down on the wheel.
Exhale: Hold the position and relax.
Inhale: Move the hands past the neck and grasp the wheel/lay the forearms on
the floor.
Exhale: Hold the position and relax.

BACKBEND FOR THE HIP FLEXORS ON THE WHEEL

Difficulty Level:

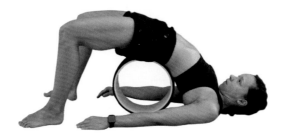

Stretches the following muscles: Hip flexors and abdominal muscles.

1. Start from the Backbend on the Wheel pose. Raise the buttocks slightly, and place the lower back completely on the wheel. Roll over the wheel, and rest the head and shoulders on the mat. The entire lower back and tailbone are in contact with the wheel.
2. Stand or stretch the legs for a more intense stretch of the hip flexors.

BREATHING
Inhale: Lift the buttocks and rest the back on the wheel.
Exhale: Roll over the wheel and rest the shoulders.
Inhale: Extend the legs.
Exhale: Hold the position and relax.

BACKBEND FOR THE HIP FLEXORS ON THE WHEEL VARIATIONS

Difficulty Level:

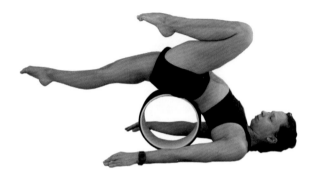

VARIATION 1

1. From the Backbend for the Hip Flexors on the Wheel pose, bend one leg and pull it to the chest.
2. Keep the hips parallel. The other leg remains in the air and actively pulls away from the center of the body to stretch the hip.

BREATHING
Inhale: Bend the leg and pull it toward the chest.
Exhale: Hold the position and relax.

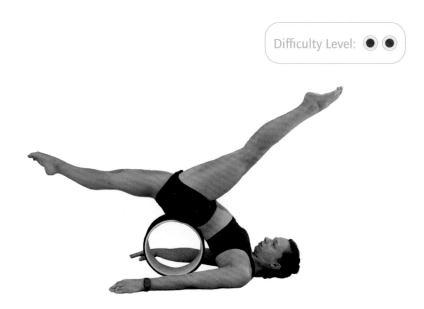

Difficulty Level: ● ●

VARIATION 2

Stretches the following areas: Back of the thigh, calves, and hip flexors.

1. From the Backbend for the Hip Flexors on the Wheel pose, stretch the bent leg and pull it to the chest. The hands remain on the ground to aid balance.
2. The other leg remains in the air and pulls in the opposite direction to the ground.
3. Try to keep the hips parallel.

BREATHING
Inhale: Extend the leg and pull it in toward the chest, and at the same time, pull the other leg to the floor.
Exhale: Hold the position and relax.

Difficulty Level: ● ● ●

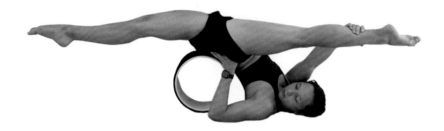

VARIATION 3

Stretches the following muscles: Back of the thigh, calves, and hip flexors.

1. Start from the Backbend for the Hip Flexors on the wheel and move directly into open splits. Bend the same arm as the leg that is pulled toward the chest and place the bent arm onto the floor. Bring hand to hip/buttocks.
2. Balance first. The body's center of gravity is on the center of the wheel. If balance is sufficient, the center of gravity can be shifted slightly to the hand. The challenge here is not to fall off the wheel.
3. Now grasp the front leg at the calf with the other hand and pull toward the center of the body. Slowly stretch the leg.
4. Maintain the pull on the leg while the other leg pulls toward the ground.
5. The exercise can be performed with the hips closed or open.

BREATHING
Inhale: Place one hand at the hip and grasp the calf from the outside with the other hand.
Exhale: Balance.
Inhale: Slowly straighten the bent leg.
Exhale: Balance, hold position and relax.

STRADDLE WITH BACKBEND ON THE WHEEL

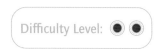

Difficulty Level:

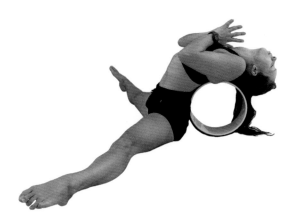

Stretches the following muscles: Back of the thigh, inner thigh, calf, abdominal muscles, chest muscles, and shoulder muscles.

1. Start in a straddle and place the wheel on the lower back.
2. Rest the upper back on the wheel, and raise the arms above the head.
3. If sufficiently flexible, grasp the wheel at neck level to intensify the stretch in the front of the upper body.

BREATHING
Inhale: Slowly lay down on the wheel and grasp it level with the neck.
Exhale: Hold position and relax.

COBRA ON THE WHEEL

Difficulty Level: ◉

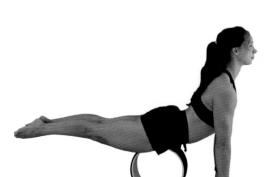

Stretches the following muscles: Chest muscles, shoulder muscles, and abdominal muscles.

1. Start in a kneeling position and open the legs slightly. Place the wheel between the legs and rest the pubic bone on the wheel.
2. Lean the body forward and bring the hands to the floor.
3. With the pubic bone, apply pressure on the wheel, and press into the floor with the hands to open the chest.
4. Easier variation: place hands on yoga blocks.
5. Release the legs from the floor and tense the glutes and legs.

BREATHING
Inhale: Lie down on the wheel and open the upper body.
Exhale: Hold the position and relax.

CHESTSTAND ON THE WHEEL II

Difficulty Level: ● ●

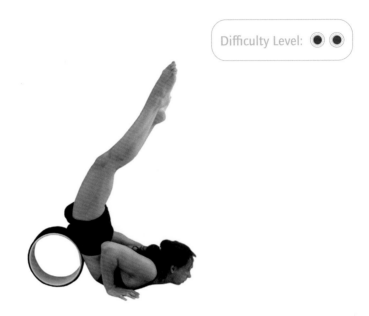

Strengthens the following muscles: Gluteal muscles, leg muscles, lower back muscles, arm and chest muscles.
Stretches the following muscles: Abdominal muscles and hip flexors.

1. From the Cobra on the Wheel pose, bend the arms, and rest the chest on the floor. At the same time, bend the legs and rest them on the wheel.
2. If the chest does not yet reach to the floor, a yoga block can be placed under the chest as an elevation.
3. The arms come to rest at the sides next to the chest and press into the floor toward the wheel. The head faces straight ahead.
4. Slowly release the legs from the wheel and lift toward the ceiling. The pubic bone is released so that only the abdomen is on the wheel.
5. The entire musculature remains tense while practicing the exercise.

BREATHING
Inhale: From the cobra, slowly place the chest on the floor.
Exhale: Balance.
Inhale: Slowly raise the legs to the ceiling.
Exhale: Hold the position and relax.

SCORPION ON THE WHEEL

Difficulty Level: ● ● ●

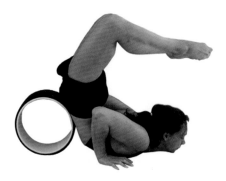

Strengthens the following muscles: Gluteal muscles, leg muscles, lower back muscles, arm and chest muscles.
Stretches the following muscles: Abdominal muscles and hip flexor.

1. From the Chest Stand on the Wheel pose, slowly bend the legs and pull them forward toward the head.
2. Press the hands into the floor to maintain contact with the wheel.
3. The entire torso muscles, as well as the gluteal muscles, are tight.

BREATHING
Inhale: Slowly lift the legs and pull them toward the head.
Exhale: Hold the position and relax.

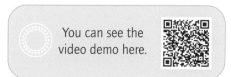

You can see the video demo here.

BRIDGE WITH THE WHEEL

Difficulty Level: ● ●

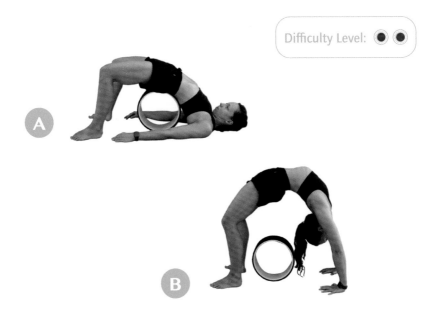

Stretches the following muscles: Abdominal and chest muscles, anterior shoulder muscles, forearms, and hip flexors.

Activates the following muscles: Leg muscles, gluteal muscles, all back muscles, and arm muscles.

1. From the Backbend for the Hip Flexors on the Wheel pose, lift both legs back up so that the knee joints are at a 90-degree angle (photo *a*).
2. Place the hands next to the ears with the fingers pointing to the feet.
3. Tighten the glutes as well as the lower back muscles, and push up the body from the arms (photo *b*). If performed cleanly, the wheel will not move.
4. Press out from the shoulders and keep the feet stable on the ground.
5. To come out of the pose, bend the arms and legs and rest the back on the wheel. Then roll down.

BREATHING
Inhale: Press up into the wheel.
Exhale: Hold the position and relax.

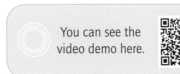

You can see the video demo here.

BRIDGE WITH THE WHEEL VARIATIONS

Difficulty Level:

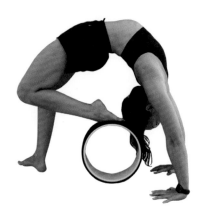

VARIATION 1

1. With sufficient body balance, try to place the foot on the wheel and push it a little toward the head.
2. To get out of this pose, follow the instructions in step 5 of the previous pose, Bridge With the Wheel, or pull the wheel out with the foot forward for a direct supine position.

BREATHING
Inhale: Place foot on wheel.
Exhale: Hold the position and relax.

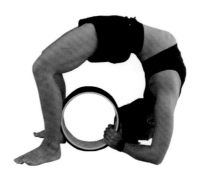

VARIATION 2

1. From the Bridge With the Wheel pose, with sufficient shoulder mobility, place the forearms on the mat to get into a forearm Bridge.
2. Attempt to grasp the wheel.
3. With good shoulder mobility, the knee joints can be extended and the feet pressed into the floor.

BREATHING
Inhale: Straighten the legs.
Exhale: Hold the position and relax.

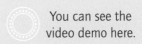

You can see the video demo here.

CAMEL WITH THE YOGA WHEEL

Difficulty Level: ● ● ●

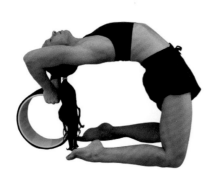

Strengthens the following muscles: Leg muscles, gluteal muscles, all back muscles, and arm muscles.

Stretches the following muscles: Abdominal, chest, shoulder muscles, hip flexor, and front of thigh.

1. Start in a kneeling position, open the legs a little more, and let the feet rotate inward slightly.
2. Grasp the wheel and hold it in front of the chest.
3. Slowly bend the lumbar spine backward, vertebra by vertebra, with the gluteal muscles permanently tensed.
4. Extend the arms as the thoracic spine flexes, and place the wheel on the floor below the head.
5. The head can be placed on the wheel for relief.
6. Move the hands in a controlled manner further and further back toward the buttocks and try to strengthen the Backbend.

BREATHING

Inhale: Activate gluteal muscles.
Exhale: Hold position.
Inhale: Bring lumbar spine into Backbend.
Exhale: Hold position.
Inhale: Flex the thoracic spine backward.
Exhale: Hold position.
Inhale: Extend arms and lower the wheel over the head to the floor.
Exhale: Hold position.
Inhale: Hands move along the wheel toward the buttocks.
Exhale: Hold position.

 You can see the video demo here.

CAMEL WITH FEET ON THE YOGA WHEEL

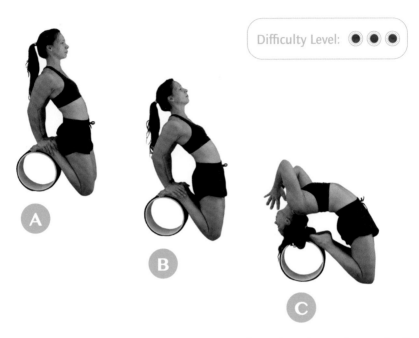

Difficulty Level: ● ● ●

Strengthens the following muscles: Leg muscles, gluteal muscles, and all back muscles.

Stretches the following muscles: Front of thighs, hip flexors, and abdominal muscles; with head down: chest muscles.

1. Start in a kneeling position and place the wheel at foot level.
2. Place the hands in front of the body and the insteps of both feet on the wheel.
3. Walk slowly with the hands toward the knees and straighten the upper body. If necessary, use a yoga block to help.
4. Place the hands on the wheel for better stability (photo *a*).
5. Tighten the buttocks and thigh muscles and push the hips forward (photo *b*).
6. Increase: Release the hands from the wheel and move into a Backbend in the spine (photo *c*). The hips continue to actively push forward.

BREATHING

Inhale: Place feet on the wheel.
Exhale: Slowly straighten up and place the hands on the wheel.
Inhale: Push hips forward or Backbend in spine.
Exhale: Hold and relax.

BOW POSE WITH THE YOGA WHEEL

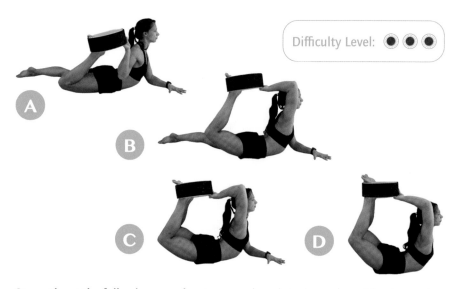

Difficulty Level: ● ● ●

Strengthens the following muscles: Leg muscles, gluteal muscles, all back muscles, and arm muscles.

Stretches the following muscles: Abdominal and chest muscles, anterior shoulder muscles, and anterior thigh muscles.

1. Line in a prone position and grasp the wheel from the outside.
2. Place one foot inside the wheel, and turn the wheel so that the opening points downward.
3. Depending on flexibility, the following positions are possible:
   a. One foot in the wheel and elbow pointing back (photo *a*).
      The front arm can be supported on the hand or forearm.
   b. The elbow can be brought forward via shoulder rotation (photo *b*).
      The front arm can be supported on the hand or forearm.
   c. In options a and b, the other foot can also be placed in the wheel (photo *c*).
   d. The hand that is on the floor can be guided to the wheel (photo *d*).
      This is also possible with both shoulder positions.
4. In all variations it is especially important that the buttocks are tight to relieve some pressure on the lower back and to build up strength.
5. Once the feet and arms are in place, the insteps of the feet push into the wheel, and the legs and arms pull upward. The chest lifts off the floor.

BREATHING
Inhale: Feet push into the wheel. At the same time, push the legs and arms up.
Exhale: Balance.

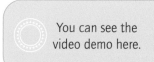
You can see the video demo here.

FLYING COBRA ON THE WHEEL

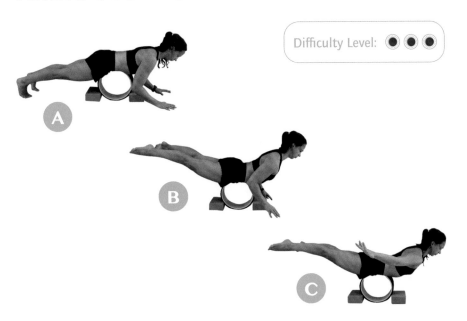

Difficulty Level: ● ● ●

Strengthens the following muscles: Lower back muscles, gluteal muscles, all leg muscles, and active chest opening.

1. Fix the Yoga Wheel between two yoga blocks.
2. Rest the abdomen on the wheel. The pubic bone presses against the wheel with the help of a pelvic tilt.
3. The hands initially remain on the floor, and the chest opens (photo *a*).
4. The feet release from the floor and the buttocks tighten (photo *b*).
5. First release one hand from the floor and bring it to the side of the body. Later, the second hand can also be released from the floor.
6. Then balance on only the lower part of the abdomen, and keep the tension in the upper body (photo *c*).

BREATHING
Inhale: Release feet from the floor.
Exhale: Pause and balance.
Inhale: Bring arms to the sides of the body.
Exhale: Hold position and balance.

COBRA WITH ONE FOOT GRIPPED OR BOW POSE

Difficulty Level: ● ● ●

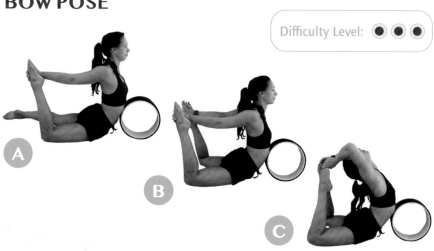

Strengthens the following muscles: Gluteal muscles, lower back muscles, and arm muscles.
Stretches the following muscles: Abdominal and chest muscles.

1. Start in a half Cobra and place the wheel in front of the body.
2. Pull the wheel toward the abdomen with one hand and place it on top.
3. Place the hands on the inside of the wheel and run them backward into a Backbend.
4. The pubic bone remains on the floor and the buttocks tense throughout the exercise.
5. Variations:
    a. Grasp one foot with the same hand from the inside (photo *a*). Bring the shoulders parallel again. Hands press against feet, feet push back.
    b. Grasp both feet with hands (photo *b*). Shoulders are aligned forward. Hands press against feet, and the feet push back.
    c. Grasp both feet with hands, and rotate elbow forward and up over by rotating the shoulder (photo *c*).

BREATHING
Inhale: Upper body straightens into a Backbend.
Exhale: Balance.
Inhale: Grasp foot or feet.
Exhale: Straighten shoulders back to front.
Inhale: Hands push into feet and feet push back. Or for step c, elbows pull upward.
Exhale: Hold and relax.

BRIDGE WITH ONE FOOT ON THE YOGA WHEEL

Difficulty Level: ● ● ●

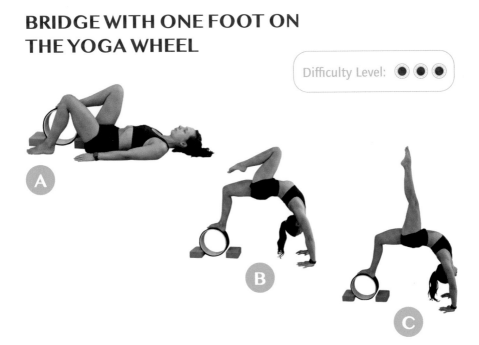

Strengthens the following muscles: Gluteal muscles, lower back muscles, shoulder muscles, and arm muscles.
Stretches the following muscles: Abdominal muscles, chest muscles, and hip flexors.

1. Fix the Yoga Wheel between two yoga blocks.
2. Start in a supine position and place one foot centrally on the Yoga Wheel (photo *a*).
3. Either stay on the shoulders or place the hands next to the ears and move into a Bridge (photo *b*).
4. Press into the wheel with the foot that is on the wheel to create basic tension in the thigh muscles.
5. Slowly lift the free leg and stretch it upward (photo *c*).
6. During the entire exercise, the gluteal muscles remain tense.

BREATHING
Inhale: Push up into shoulder Bridge or normal Bridge.
Exhale: Balance.
Inhale: Slowly lift the free leg.
Exhale: Balance.

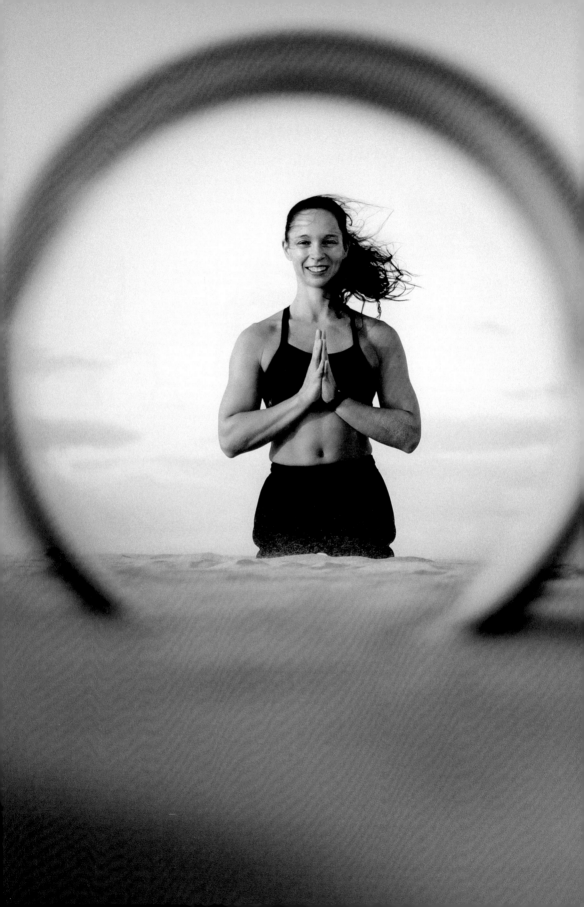

FORWARD BENDS
AND HIP OPENERS

CHILD'S POSE WITH THE WHEEL

Difficulty Level:

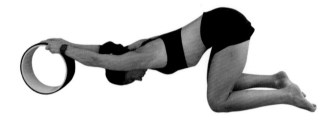

Stretches the following muscles: Chest, shoulder, and upper back muscles.

1. Bring the knees hip width apart, and place the hands on the wheel.
2. Roll forward with the wheel until the torso and hips form a 90-degree angle. The knees are under the hips.
3. Actively pull the shoulders forward using the hands. Keep the back straight and pull in the belly button.

BREATHING
Inhale: Place hands on the wheel and roll forward.
Exhale: Hold position and relax.

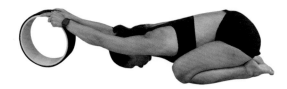

VARIATION 1

1. To intensify the stretch, lower the upper body and stretch the chest muscles.
    Avoid a hollow back.

BREATHING
Inhale: Continue lowering the upper body.
Exhale: Hold the position and relax.

KNEELING DANCER

Difficulty Level: ● ●

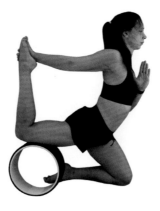

Stretches the following muscles: Hip flexor, front thigh, chest, and front shoulder muscles.

1. Start on All Fours and place the wheel next to one thigh.
2. Straighten the upper body slightly and place one thigh on the wheel. Bend the knee joint that is on the floor, and pull the buttocks toward the wheel.
3. Bend the leg that is on the wheel and grasp it from the inside with the same hand.
4. Rotate the upper body forward again to stretch the chest and shoulders.
5. Place the other hand in front of the chest and balance.
6. If it is too unstable, a yoga block can be used for support.

BREATHING
Inhale: Place thighs on the wheel.
Exhale: Straighten the upper body.
Inhale: Grasp the foot.
Exhale: Rotate upper body forward.

LUNGE TWIST

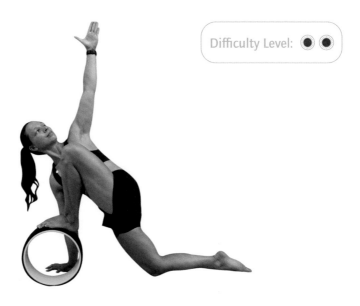

Difficulty Level: ● ●

Strengthens the following muscles: Thigh muscles.
Stretches the following muscles: Hip flexors, front and anterior thigh, and lateral trunk muscles.

1. Start in a knee Lunge and carefully place one foot on the wheel.
    Roll forward a bit more if needed.
2. Bring the hips forward, and place the opposite hand on the floor or on
    a yoga block if the wheel is too high.
3. Turn the chest toward the thigh and pull the other arm toward the ceiling.

BREATHING
Inhale: Place the foot on the wheel and place the hand on the floor/block in position.
Exhale: Turn the chest toward the thigh.

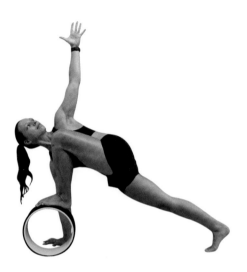

VARIATION 1

1. When completely stable, release the back knee from the floor and straighten the leg.
2. Bring the hip forward and place the opposite hand on the floor or yoga block if the wheel is too high.
3. Turn the chest to the thigh and pull the arm to the ceiling.

BREATHING

Inhale: Place the foot on the wheel and place the hand on the floor/block in position.

Exhale: Turn the chest toward the thigh. Release the knee from the floor.

LUNGE WITH BACKBEND

Difficulty Level: ● ●

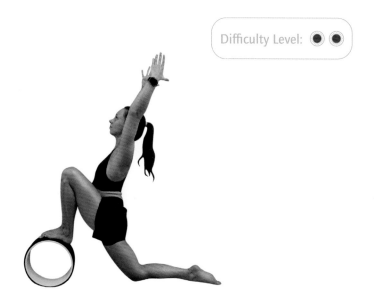

Strengthens the following muscles: Thigh, gluteal, and lower back muscles.
Stretches the following muscles: Hip flexors, front of thighs, and chest muscles.

1. Start in the lunge position with one knee on the floor and one foot on the wheel.
2. Push the hip forward. Make sure the knee on the wheel is not pushed over the top of the foot.
3. Keep the hip bones parallel.
4. If you feel stable, bring the arms up over the side, lower the shoulder blades, and open the chest muscles using a small Backbend.
5. Actively tense the buttocks and lower back muscles.

BREATHING
Inhale: Put the foot down on the wheel and push the hips forward.
Exhale: Bring the arms above the head.
Inhale: Open the chest.
Exhale: Hold the position and relax.

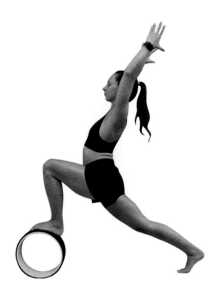

VARIATION 1

1.   For increasing the sense of balance, the back leg can be stretched.

BREATHING
Inhale: Put the foot down on the wheel, straighten the back knee, and push the hips forward.
Exhale: Bring the arms above the head.
Inhale: Open the chest.
Exhale: Hold the position and relax.

LONG BALANCE LUNGE

Difficulty Level: ● ●

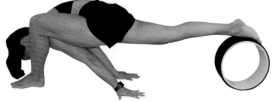

Strengthens the following muscles: Thigh and gluteal muscles.
Stretches the following muscles: Hip flexors and front of the thighs.

1. Start on All Fours and place the wheel between the legs.
2. Place one foot between the hands and rest the back foot on the wheel.
   Make sure the front knee joint is over the heel.
3. Roll backward with the wheel until the leg is extended.
4. Tighten the toes to hold the wheel.
5. The hands can be placed as follows:
6. Both hands can move to the same side as the stretched leg and remain in position.
   a. The hands can slide level with the buttocks, and the arms can be stretched.
   b. The hands can be placed on the bent leg and the upper body straightened.
7. Actively push the hips to the floor.

BREATHING
Inhale: From All Fours, bring one foot forward between the hands.
Exhale: Place the other foot on the wheel and roll backward.
Inhale: Push the hips toward the floor.
Exhale: Hold the position and relax.

HAMSTRING STRETCH

Difficulty Level: ●

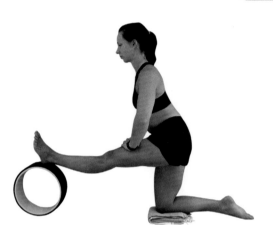

Stretches the following muscles: Back of the thigh.

1. Start in a lunge position with knees on the ground, and carefully place one heel on the wheel.
2. Slowly roll the heel along the wheel until the leg is extended.
3. Straighten the torso and tilt the pelvis forward slightly to intensify the stretch in the hip flexor.
4. Keep the hip bones parallel.
5. Intensify the stretch in the back of the thigh by applying pressure to the wheel with the heel.

BREATHING
Inhale: Place the heel on the wheel and roll forward.
Exhale: Straighten the upper body and tilt the pelvis forward.
Inhale: Put pressure on the wheel and stretch the back of the thigh.
Exhale: Hold the position and relax.

SPLITS ON THE WHEEL

Difficulty Level: ● ● ●

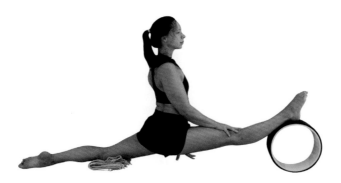

Stretches the following muscles: Back of the thigh, gluteal muscles, and hip flexors.

1. From the Thigh Back Stretch, slowly roll the wheel forward to stretch the back leg.
2. If the wheel is too high at the beginning, support the hands on two yoga blocks for stabilization.
3. Try to keep the hips and shoulders parallel, even if the hips life up a bit at the start.

BREATHING
Inhale: Roll forward with the wheel to stretch the back leg.
Exhale: Hold the position and relax.

HAMSTRING STRETCH VARIATIONS

Difficulty Level: ● ●

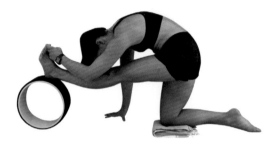

VARIATION 1

1. Grasp the big toe with the same hand as the extended leg and actively pull the foot.
2. The pelvis remains tilted forward to maintain the stretch in the hip flexor. The hip bones remain at one level.

BREATHING
Inhale: Grasp the big toe and actively pull the foot in.
Exhale: Hold the position and relax.

VARIATION 2

1. Lean the upper body vertebra by vertebra toward the extended leg.
2. Hands remain on the floor for stabilization.
3. The hips remain closed.

BREATHING
Inhale: Lean the upper body forward.
Exhale: Hold the position and relax.

TUCK ON THE WHEEL

Difficulty Level: ⦿

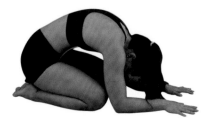

Stretches the following muscles: No mandatory stretching—the primary focus is on pulling the vertebrae apart one by one and relaxing the spine.

1. Start in a kneeling position and sit on the calves. Open the legs a little and place the wheel between the legs.
2. Lift the chest and pull the abdomen in. Rest the abdomen on the wheel.
3. Start at the top of the rib cage and curve the back, vertebra by vertebra, until the rib cage is completely resting on the wheel.
4. Rest the arms either around the wheel or on the floor.

BREATHING
Inhale: Lift the chest and slowly place it on the wheel.
Exhale: When the final position is reached, relax, and direct the exhalation to the spine.

SITTING FORWARD BEND ON THE WHEEL

Difficulty Level: ◉

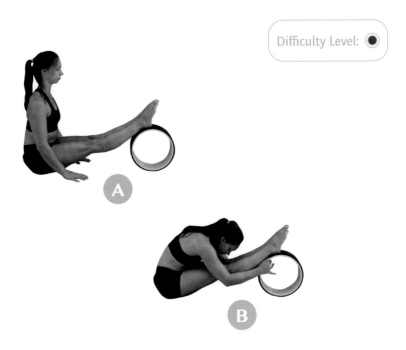

Stretches the following muscles: Back extensors, back of the thighs, and calves.

1. Start in a seated position and place the wheel in front of the legs.
2. Place the feet in the center of the wheel and hold it at the edges.
3. Actively pull the chest up so that the back becomes straight and the stretch in the back of the thighs intensifies (photo *a*).
4. To further increase intensity, lean the upper body forward toward the legs (photo *b*). The wheel can be gripped at the edge.
5. The exercise can be performed with a straight or curved back.

BREATHING
Inhale: Place the legs on the wheel and grasp the inner edge with the hands.
Exhale: Straighten the upper body.
Inhale: Lean forward with a straight back.
Exhale: Hold the position and relax.

SITTING FORWARD BEND WITH ONE LEG ON THE WHEEL

Difficulty Level:

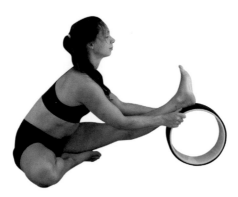

Stretches the following muscles: Back of the thigh, inner thigh, and calves.

1. Start in a seated position and place the wheel in front of the legs.
2. Angle one leg and rest the other on the wheel.
3. The hip bones remain parallel.
4. Hold on to the wheel and extend the chest so that the back stretches.

BREATHING
Inhale: Place one leg on the wheel and grasp the wheel.
Exhale: Raise the upper body so that the back remains straight.

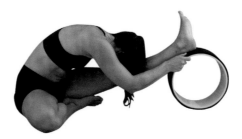

VARIATION 1

1. To intensify the stretch, pull on the wheel with the hands (possibly bending the arms), and lean the upper body further forward.
2. The back may become curved.

BREATHING
Inhale: Pull on the wheel and lean the upper body toward the wheel.
Exhale: Hold the position and relax.

LUNGE WITH THE WHEEL

Difficulty Level: ◉

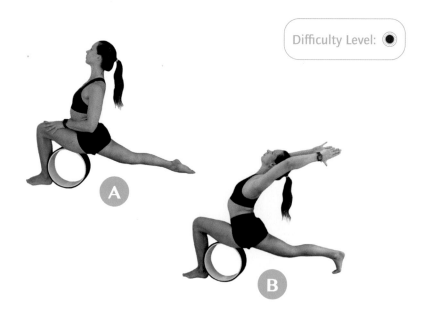

Stretches the following muscles: Hip flexors, front of the thigh, abdominal muscles, and shoulder muscles.

1. Start in a kneeling position and place the wheel in front. Place one foot in front of the wheel. Make sure the knee is at a 90-degree angle and under the heel.
2. Move the other leg back while pushing the hip forward (photo *a*).
3. The back of the thigh of the front leg now rests on the wheel, which presses against the front calf.
4. If stable enough, the back leg can be stretched over the instep or toe of the foot.
5. Bringing the arms up over the side, activate the glutes as well as lower back muscles, and move into a slight Backbend (photo *b*).
6. Open the chest toward the ceiling.
7. The shoulders remain pulled low during the Backbend.

BREATHING
Inhale: Put the weight on the wheel.
Exhale: Raise the arms to the sides.
Inhale: Bend backward.
Exhale: Hold the position and relax.

PIGEON ON THE WHEEL WITH FOOT GRASP

Difficulty Level:

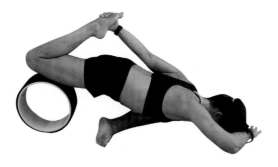

Stretches the following muscles: Hip flexors, gluteal muscles, and front of the thighs.

1. Start from the Kneeling Dancer pose and place both hands on the floor.
2. Pull the leg forward on the floor and return the lower leg to a 45-degree angle.
3. The leg on the wheel can remain extended or actively bent and pulled toward the buttocks.
4. Slowly lean the upper body forward. Either stay on the hands or switch to the forearms.
5. If sufficiently flexible, the back foot can be grasped with the opposite hand.
6. More difficult variation: position the front lower leg so that the knee joint is at a 90-degree angle.

BREATHING
Inhale: Place hands on the floor.
Exhale: Place lower leg on the floor and rest the upper body if necessary.
Inhale: Bend back leg and grasp foot.
Exhale: Hold the stretch.

PIGEON WITH THE WHEEL

Difficulty Level: ◉

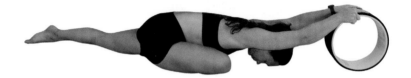

Stretches the following muscles: Hip flexors, gluteal muscles, and chest muscles.
Activates the following areas: Shoulder muscles.

1. Start from All Fours with one leg forward at a 45-degree angle.
    The thigh and the outside of the calf are on the floor.
2. Either place the back leg to the side at a 90-degree angle or
    extend it backward on the hip line.
3. Press the hands into the floor and lift the pelvis briefly to bring
    the hips into the correct position. Make sure the hip bones are in line
    with each other.
4. Place the wheel in front of the front leg and rest the hands on it.
    Slowly roll forward while inhaling.
5. Keep the hips closed throughout the exercise.

BREATHING
Inhale: From all fours, position the leg in front.
Exhale: Bring the hip bones forward.
Inhale: Slowly roll the wheel forward.
Exhale: Hold the position and relax.

STRADDLE WITH FORWARD BEND

Difficulty Level: ● ●

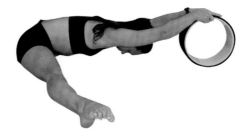

Stretches the following muscles: Inner thigh, back of the thigh, calves, gluteal muscles, and chest muscles.
Activates the following areas: Shoulder muscles.

1. Start in a seated position and open the legs into a straddle.
2. Place the wheel in front of the body and rest the hands on it.
3. Straighten the upper body.
4. The buttocks actively pull back. Moved the lower back into a slightly hollowed position.
5. Slowly roll forward with the wheel and hands. Make sure the back stays in the starting position.

BREATHING
Inhale: Start in a straddle position and place the hands on the wheel.
Exhale: Straighten the upper body. The back assumes a slightly hollowed position.
Inhale: Walk forward with the wheel.
Exhale: Hold the position and relax.

ONE-LEG SUMO SQUAT

Difficulty Level: ● ●

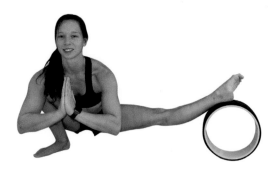

Strengthens the following muscles: Abdominal and back muscles.
Stretches the following muscles: Back of the thigh, inner thigh, hip flexor, and gluteal muscles.

1. Place the wheel sideways at hip level and move into a squat position.
2. Using the floor as support, extend the leg near the wheel, and rest the heel on the wheel. Bend the standing leg so that the knee is under the foot.
3. Sink the buttocks lower to the floor, and bring the hands in front of the chest into a prayer position.
4. Straighten the chest and bring the back into an upright position.

BREATHING
Inhale: Lower the buttocks to the floor and straighten the chest.
Exhale: Hold the position and relax.

FORWARD BEND WITH THE WHEEL

Difficulty Level: ⦿

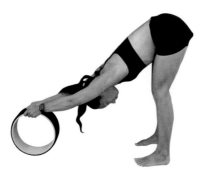

Stretches the following muscles: Back of the thighs, calves, and gluteal muscles.

1. Place the feet hip width apart and place the wheel in front of the feet.
2. The upper body bends forward with the back straight and the belly button pulled in.
3. Place both hands on the wheel and, while inhaling, pull the spine in a lengthwise direction by rolling the wheel forward.
4. Actively pull the buttocks up and extend the knee joints.
5. Use breathing to build length in the spine and back of the thighs.

BREATHING
Inhale: The upper body leans forward and the hands pull forward.
Exhale: Pull the shoulders back again and sink lower with the upper body.

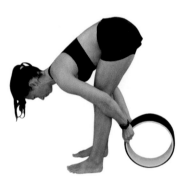

VARIATION 1

1. To intensify the hamstring back stretch, place the wheel behind the heels and hold it over the outside of the rim.
2. Actively press it into the floor and bring the upper body closer to the thighs.
3. At the same time, open the chest and extend the back again.

BREATHING
Inhale: The upper body leans forward and the hands push into the wheel.
Exhale: Pull the shoulders back again, pull on the wheel, and sink lower with the upper body.

TWO-LEG DOG WITH THE WHEEL

Difficulty Level: ● ●

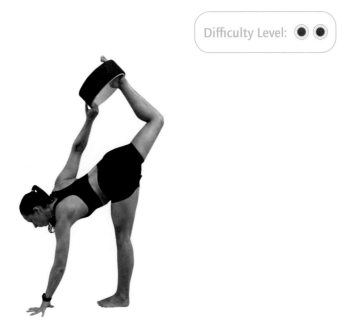

Strengthens the following muscles: Abdominal muscles and back muscles.
Stretches the following areas: Back of the thigh, calf, hip flexor, and chest muscles.

1. Start in a standing position and grasp the wheel from the outside.
   Place the corresponding foot on the inside of the wheel.
2. Tilt forward from the center of the body and bring the free hand to the floor.
3. Point the tips of the toes toward the shin to lock the wheel in place.
   The associated knee joint remains bent.
4. The hand that is on the wheel pulls the bent leg diagonally toward the
   other shoulder so that the hip opens more.

BREATHING

Inhale: Place the foot on the inside of the wheel.
Exhale: Tilt forward and place the free hand on the floor.
Inhale: Pull the wheel diagonally to the other shoulder.
Exhale: Hold the position and relax.

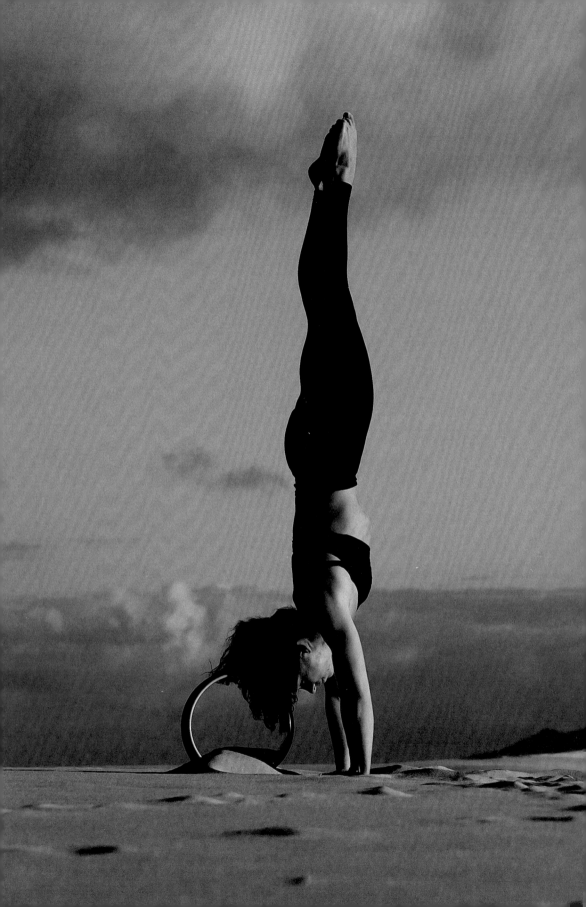

REVERSE POSES

PLOW ON THE WHEEL

Difficulty Level: ● ●

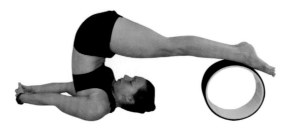

Stretches the following muscles: Neck muscles, upper and lower back muscles, gluteal muscles, and back of the thighs.

1. Start in the supine position and hold the wheel over the head.
2. Lift the buttocks and rest the insteps of both feet on the wheel.
3. The hands lie next to the body or grip the floor behind the back for additional stabilization.
4. Push the wheel backward with the instep of the feet until the buttocks are above the shoulders.

BREATHING
Inhale: The buttocks lift off the mat, and the insteps of the feet are placed on the wheel. Either clasp the hands or leave them beside the body.
Exhale: Balance.
Inhale: Continue moving the insteps of the feet until the buttocks are slowly over the shoulders.
Exhale: Hold the position.

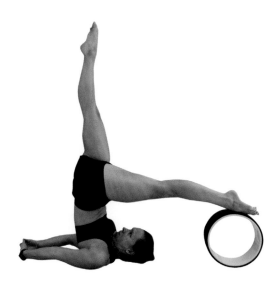

VARIATION 1

1. Alternately lift one leg to the ceiling and balance on the wheel with one foot instep.

BREATHING

Inhale: The buttocks lift off the mat, and the insteps of the feet are placed on the wheel. Either clasp the hands or leave them beside the body.

Exhale: Balance.

Inhale: Continue moving the insteps of the feet until the buttocks are slowly over the shoulders.

Exhale: Hold the position and relax or lift one leg to the ceiling.

BENT-LEG PLOW ON THE WHEEL

Difficulty Level: ● ● ●

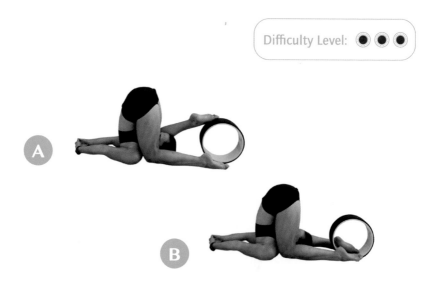

Stretches the following muscles: Neck muscles, upper and lower back muscles, and gluteal muscles.

1. The starting pose is the Plow on the Wheel.
2. From there, release one foot instep from the wheel and bend the knee joint. Slowly, and while inhaling, place the leg to the ear or shoulder (photo *a*).
3. Alternate bending the legs and placing them back on the wheel.
4. If the flexibility is good, both feet can be released from the wheel and placed on the floor (photo *b*). Bend the knee joints farther while inhaling, bring them to the ear or shoulder, and then place them on the floor.

BREATHING
Inhale: Release one instep from the wheel, bend the associated knee and pull it toward the ear or shoulder.
Exhale: Hold the position and relax.
Inhale: Place the instep back on the wheel.
Exhale: Shift the weight and prepare to change sides.

HEADSTAND BALANCE WITH KNEES ON THE WHEEL

Difficulty Level: ● ● ●

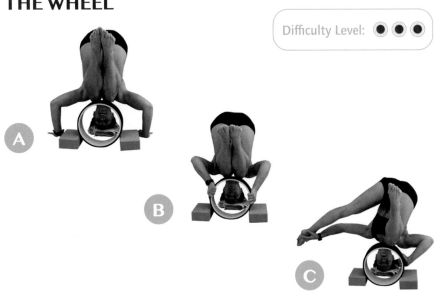

Strengthens the following muscles: All back, abdominal, and leg muscles.

1. Start in a kneeling position and place the wheel with the opening in front of the knees.
2. Place the hands at the sides over the wheel.
3. Place your feet on the floor and rest the head half a hand's width on the floor.
4. Now place both knees on the wheel and pull the feet toward the buttocks (photo *a*).
5. Balance with the knees on the wheel (photo *b*).
6. Pull the buttocks to head height and maintain the tension in the back.
7. With the hands, reach over the shoulder and press into the floor, and hold this tension.
8. Increase:
   a. Bring the hands to the wheel and grip around the edge of the wheel.
   b. Release one knee from the wheel and pull it outward, grasping it with the same hand (photo *c*).

BREATHING
Breathe normally during the entire practice.

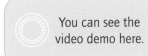
You can see the video demo here.

FOREARM STAND WITH THE WHEEL

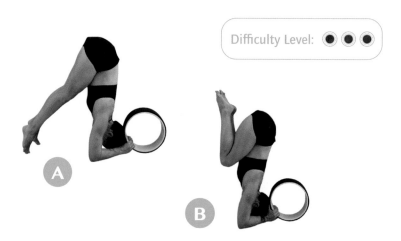

Difficulty Level: ● ● ●

A

B

Strengthens the following muscles: Shoulder muscles, chest and back muscles, and abdominal muscles.

1. Start by placing the wheel against a wall or yoga block.
2. Place the forearms on the mat and grasp the wheel with the hands.
    At the same time, press the back of the head against the wheel.
3. Walk forward with the feet until the buttocks are above the head (photo *a*).
4. There are three options for the leg position:
    a. Place two yoga blocks wider than hip width under the feet.
        This makes it easier to lift the legs at the start (beginner; photo *b*).
    b. Place a yoga block in the middle and far enough away so that the
        legs can still be stretched (intermediate).
    c. Start directly without a yoga block in the closed leg position (advanced).
5. Tilt the pelvis slightly forward to activate the abdominal muscles and lock
    the lower back. At the same time, press into the floor over the forearms.
    This will squeeze out and activate the shoulders.
6. Lift the legs.
7. The head can either:
    a. Continue to be pressed against the wheel for added stability
        (beginner and intermediate).
    b. Hang freely between the wheel and the ground (advanced).
8. At the beginning, no matter which leg position is chosen, the legs
    are bent and pulled to the chest.
9. For intermediate/advanced, after balancing the legs, there is the
    possibility of slowly stretching the legs to the ceiling. While straightening,
    make sure to maintain tension in the buttocks.

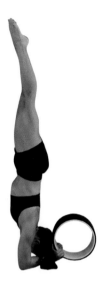

ANOTHER ALTERNATIVE

1. Without a yoga block, start directly with one leg in the air and lift
    the other leg using the pelvic tilt (advanced).
2. Be careful not to fall into a hollow back but to keep the pelvis actively
    tilted to maintain tension in the center of the body.

BREATHING
Inhale: Press the forearms and shoulders into the floor.
Exhale: Release the legs from the floor.
With regular breathing, either keep the legs in a small tuck or stretch them out.

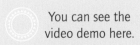
You can see the video demo here.

HEADSTAND TO FLIP ON THE WHEEL

Difficulty Level: ● ● ●

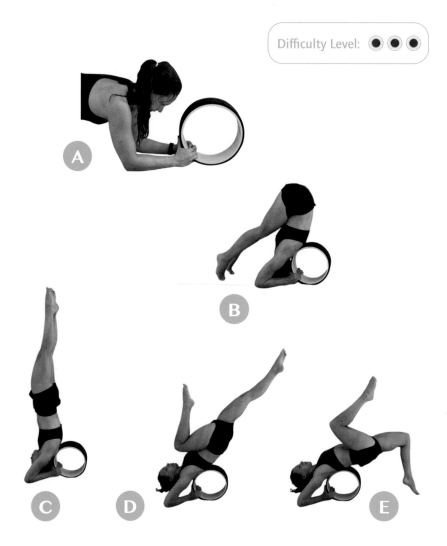

Strengthens the following muscles: All back, abdominal, gluteal, and leg muscles.

1. Start in a kneeling position and place the wheel in front of the body (photo *a*). Lean on the forearms and place the hands as follows:
   a. Little finger is under the wheel.
   b. Ring finger, middle finger, and index finger are on the inside of the wheel.
   c. The thumb is on the outside of the wheel.

2. Place the head on the floor about half a hand's width away, press the forearms into the floor, and straighten the knees and lift the buttocks (photo *b*).
3. Walk the feet forward and rest the shoulders on the wheel.
4. Using the strength in the arms, press the wheel into the ground so it is fixed.
5. One at a time, lift the legs by activating the abdominal muscles and initially try to pause in a tuck position.
6. After that, the legs can either:
    a. Be positioned in a straddle.
    b. Be stretched upward into a headstand (photo *c*).
7. Avoid a hollow back and try to activate the abdominal and lower back muscles.
8. From the Headstand position, bend and pull one leg toward the chest and extend the other behind (photo *d*).
9. The shoulder remains on the wheel. Now shift the weight further forward so the rest of the thoracic spine is on the wheel.
10. Maintain tension in the arms and, with the hands, pull even harder on the wheel to fix it to the back.
11. The extended leg is placed on the floor, and the rest of the spine is placed on the wheel (photo *e*). Important: Do not let go of the wheel with the hands!

BREATHING
Inhale: Lift legs off the floor to go into the Headstand.
Exhale: Balance.
Inhale: Legs into straddle or full headstand.
Exhale: Balance.
Inhale: Bring the rest of the thoracic spine on the wheel.
Exhale: Put the leg down on the floor.

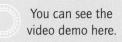 You can see the video demo here.

KNEE-ARM BALANCE

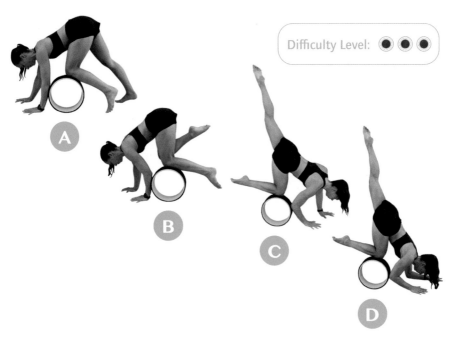

Difficulty Level: ● ● ●

Strengthens the following muscles: All back and abdominal muscles.

1. Start in a Downward Dog. The wheel is on one side.
2. Place the lower part of the knee and the same elbow on the wheel.
   Push into the wheel with the knee and lift the foot from the floor.
   Press the elbow into the wheel (photo *a*).
3. Shift the weight to both hands and slowly lift the free leg from the mat (photo *b*).
4. Balance out and extend the leg upward, maintaining balance (photo *c*).
5. Maintain tension throughout the center of the body and balance out.
6. Easier variation: Fix the wheel with two yoga blocks.
7. Harder variation: Press the forearm of the free outside arm evenly into
   the floor to keep the shoulder parallel (photo *d*).

BREATHING
Inhale: Rest the lower part of the knee and the elbow on the wheel.
Exhale: Shift the weight to the hands
and release the back foot.
Inhale: Pull the leg up.
Exhale: Balance and maintain
the tension.

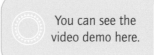 You can see the
video demo here.

INDEX

ABOUT THE AUTHOR

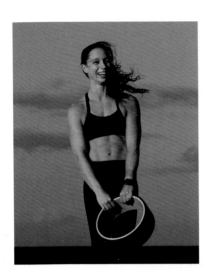

Selina Reichert was born in Frankfurt am Main (Germany) in 1994 and is a yoga and pole sports coach and Instructor. She studied fitness economics and completed her master's degree in Business Administration.

She discovered her enthusiasm for Hatha and Vinyasa Yoga in 2009 after she began using yoga and weight training as means to alleviate back pain caused by scoliosis and extreme stiffening of the lumbar spine. She started training with the Yoga Wheel in 2015. She started training with the Yoga Wheel in 2015.

For Selina, yoga is part of a good work-life balance because yoga helps her to pause and relax, even in stressful times. In order to share the positive benefits of yoga for mind and body with other people, Selina has been teaching yoga for several years since 2016. In 2018, she developed her own course format with the Yoga Wheel. The popularity with her course participants at the time prompted her to write a book about the Yoga Wheel. In 2020, she became a full-time self-employed yoga and pole trainer and founded her online studio Yoga and Pole Art by Selina. Selina has also had her own academy since 2022 and is training both pole sports trainers and Yoga Wheel trainers according to her own course concept.